Massage for Body & Soul

lates the functions of all the glands in the body. Then work on the reflexes to the thyroid, ovaries and the neck.

Inflammation: Dr. Houston has indicated that inflammation anywhere in the body can be relieved by pressing the point on the soles of the feet, about two to two-and-a-half inches from the back edge of the heel (toward the toes), in the center of the foot at the junction of the arch and the ball of the heel.

Kidney stones: The reflexes to the kidneys, pituitary, thyroid and the parathyroids.

Legs: If the legs are puffy or swollen, drain the lymphatic system by "milking" between the big and second toes (see Chapter 3, Fig. 20). Massage the reflexes to the kidneys in order to increase urination, and work on the reflex to the adrenal glands.

Liver: Work on the reflexes to the liver and the thyroid, but do not do so more frequently than twice a week. Among its many other functions, the liver stores protein; it is also directly influenced by the thyroid gland.

Lungs: Massage all five zones, on the top and the bottom of each foot. Work also on the reflexes to the bronchial tubes (Area 10). Do the wrists and the tops of the hands as well.

Lymph glands: It is, of course, important to do the milking of the glands between the big and the second toe. To reach the lymph glands in the front of the body, particularly the breasts, massage the entire top of each foot. The lymph glands in the groin may be reached through reflexes on the top of the foot from ankle to ankle.

Mental sluggishness: Massage the reflexes to the pituitary and thyroid glands, and work on the tip of the big toe.

Migraine headaches: Work on the reflexes to the solar plexus, the tip of the big toe and the cervical reflexes on the edge of the big toe. Massage the reflex to the colon if it is tender, and work also on the reflex to the coccyx. The coccyx is the bone at the base of the spinal column which is composed of four fused rudimentary vertebrae. Once again, it is a key point to many areas and organs.

Mucus: In cases of excessive mucus, do the reflexes to the ileocecal valve and to the adrenals. A malfunction of the ileocecal valve is often caused by an insuffient cortisone supply from the adrenals.

Muscle cramps: Work on the reflex to the coccyx and on the parathyroids, which are the body's calcium distributors. Muscle cramps are often caused by a lack of calcium in the muscle.

Neck: Tension and stiffness in the neck are often the result of impaired drainage of the lymphatic system, and so tension spreads to the shoulders. Work on the drainage by milking the lymphatic system. Massage the points on the vertical line nearest the second toe between the top and root of the big toe, and the root of the big toe itself. Also do the reflexes to the cervical area of the spine and those to the shoulder area. Gently rotate, or "circumduct," the big toe. You should also press directly beneath and above the collar bone.

Nervousness: Massage the reflexes to the solar plexus, and the pituitary and thyroid glands. For relaxation, you can massage these reflexes daily.

Sciatica: For pain along the sciatic nerve, start the massage from the outside edge of the left foot at a point about two-and-a-half to three inches from the heel and proceed down to about one inch from the heel. Return to the starting point and work across the foot to the spinal line at the inside edge of the foot. This is the lumbar area. At this point, change the angle and work on the spine toward the heel as far as you wish. Then massage the outside top of the foot, starting about one-and-a-half inches from the heel on the outside edge, and proceed toward the ankle bone. Press the reflexes to the hip, then move along the Achilles tendon to about two inches above the ankle. Repeat this procedure on the right foot. Work also on the reflexes to the kidneys and bladder because uric acid usually is one cause of sciatica. The colon can cause it also, so work on this reflex, as well as on the prostate gland which, if enlarged, contributes to the irritation of the sciatic nerve.

The sciatic nerve, the largest nerve in the body, starts from the sacral area and extends down to the back of the thigh, dividing there into two parts, one extending along the tibia (the inner larger bone of the leg), down to the ankle. The other part of the sciatic nerve extends along the fibula, the thin outer bone between the knee and ankle. This explains why we find reflexes to the sciatic nerve in so many places.

Shoulder Joint: Rotate the fifth toe and work on the ball beneath it. An injury to the shoulder could even affect the lumbar area, so work on that reflex, as well as on the reflexes to the shoulder blade and the neck.

Skin: If the skin is dry, discolored by a yellowish pigmentation, or if there are skin eruptions, massage the reflexes to the liver, pituitary, thyroid and the adrenals.

Sinuses: Massage the big toe and the balls of all the other toes. Do the reflex to the ileocecal valve. And if the recipient's digestion is faulty, massage the reflexes to the intestines.

It is also helpful for the sinuses to spray a mixture of one part lemon juice to three parts warm water into the nostrils twice daily. Bathing the eyes in lemon juice diluted with water in the morning and in the evening may also be helpful. Lemon possesses disinfectant qualities.

Small Intestines: Massage all five zones on each foot.

Varicose veins: Massage the reflexes to the adrenals and the parathyroids. As noted above, the adrenals regulate muscle tone. If digestion is a problem, work on the reflexes to the intestines, and on the forearms and elbows on the places that directly correspond to the affected areas on the legs. You will have to estimate the zones. Phlebitis and varicose ulcers result from both impaired circulation and (quite often) a malfunction of the colon.

Vocal cords: To strengthen the vocal cords, massage the big toe and the portion nearest the second toe. Do also the reflexes to the throat. The recipient himself can massage the sides of his nose.

Water retention: To help relieve puffiness in the extremities, massage the reflexes to the adrenals, heart and the kidneys.

Weight: If either underweight or overweight, massage the reflex to the thyroid. If there is constipation as well, work on the reflexes to the intestines.

Whiplash: Massage the reflex to the cervical area, which is on the edge of the big toe. Work on the ball of the foot, below both the big and second toe; also on the reflexes to the neck and shoulders, and rotate the big toe.

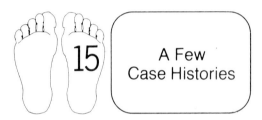

15

A Few Case Histories

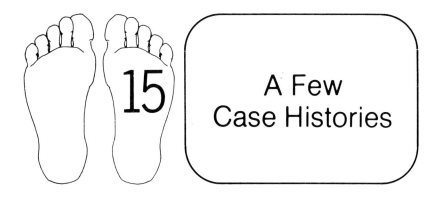

15 A Few Case Histories

It may be useful to examine several case histories that I have encountered. You will find that there are no "typical" cases. All cases that you take on require your full attention and care. And, as pointed out earlier (in Chapter 8), the masseur has a responsibility to the recipient to be as free as possible from tension and negative emotion. This is because there is a subtle exchange of feeling between the recipient and the masseur during the session. Positive and lasting results are not the result of a mere mechanical employment of the techniques. The more relaxed and clear you are about the service you perform for others, the more the session will benefit the whole person.

A man in his mid-twenties, looking thin, weak and tired, came to me for a massage. He told me that he had lost his appetite and that he was losing weight even though he was forcing himself to eat. No one had as yet been able to learn what was wrong. Following a few sessions of compression massage however, this young man was eating normally again, had noticeably more energy, and was gaining weight and strength.

Pain, stiffness of the neck and a constantly stuffed nose were the complaints of a man who said he had had the neck condition for about a year. He was not able to move his head from side to side at all, and the severely blocked nasal passages were apparent the moment he began to speak. But after a few sessions he could move his head, and his nose had cleared. "You're a healer!" he exclaimed. The "healer," I explained, is the ancient method of the body healing itself based upon a deep wisdom and knowledge of the nature of the human system.

Red spots covering the face of a woman who came to me were caused, she said, by "some kind of allergy." There was a constant itching, and she just could not keep her hands away from her face. After 20 minutes of massage the itching ceased, and after a few more sessions, it stopped altogether. I then taught her how and where to work on her feet, and instructed her to do so daily, so that she no longer required my services.

A woman in her 50's who had advanced cancer in the left breast came to me once a week for massage. Her entire left arm and hand were so swollen that they looked shapeless, and she could hardly bend the arm.

The swelling diminished markedly after each session, remaining that way for three days, during which she felt much better. But in this case, unfortunately, the improvement could not be permanent.

A certain young man kept making appointments for massage even when it seemed he did not really need them. He was healthy, but his feet were tender. After several sessions the tenderness was not nearly as pronounced, but he kept coming. I finally asked why he continued to return. He then told me that the session served as a form of psychotherapy for him: He felt relaxed for a week following each session, slept well for the first time in years, handled his problems and job with more skill, and even his memory had improved. "You have magic hands," he said.

A young woman came to me with a lump the size of a walnut in her armpit. She had been scheduled for surgery. She came to me for several sessions, after which the lump disappeared. She informed me that when she first came, she did not really believe that the problem could be helped through massage, but she had wanted to try a form of natural healing before going in for surgery. How fortunate that she did!

I often hear people make comments about their own experience with reflexology which are quite similar to the experiences of many others as well. One comment frequently heard is that after the session the recipient feels as if he or she is "walking on air," or that they feel "weightless, just like a feather." They speak of the "wave of warmth" flowing through the body, the sensation of "lightning" passing through them, or of feeling that they are "opened up" to new ideas or sensations.

Sometimes however, the results are not so spectacular. A woman in her early forties came to see if I could help her. She had suffered from rheumatoid arthritis from early childhood, was in constant pain and received cortisone injections regularly. I was extremely cautious, and worked gently on the reflexes to the solar plexus and on the big toe of each foot as well for about five minutes only. She called me later to tell me that she had been so sick the evening after receiving the massage that she could not report for work on the following day. This was, of course, a powerful purificatory reaction of her system. She returned a week later, and we both hoped that the reaction would gradually lessen in intensity. We tried it for five weeks, with no easing of the severe reactions whatsoever. Evidently, after 35 years of this chronic condition, her body had become so saturated with toxins and medication that the purification process would take a very long time. Eventually she would have been helped, but who can say how much? Since she could not afford to miss one work day a week, we decided — to our mutual regret — to forego further sessions.

A woman in her early thirties came to me crying. When I asked her what the problem was, she replied that she was perfectly healthy and she did not know exactly why she had come. But a brief interview revealed that she was upset because she was about to lose her secretarial job. She had been making so many mistakes that her boss informed her that unless she improved she would soon be fired. I was happy to learn that after a few sessions her concentration and the speed of her work had improved a great deal — to the point where she made almost no mistakes. Her boss praised her performance and even gave her a raise in salary. "You saved my job!" she said.

Another woman, weak, nervous, and afflicted with pains in the joints throughout the body, found relief for two days after the massage session, after which the pain returned. I then learned from her husband that she virtually lived on coffee and doughnuts. She drank 20 cups of coffee a day, and had doughnuts as often as five times a day! He found it necessary to cook for himself in order to get more nutritious food. My time and effort had been wasted, since she refused to change her eating habits — which actually stemmed from a mental-emotional condition. I had to stop giving her massage.

So be prepared: Some cases, for whatever reason, cannot be helped. I am not sure of the percentage of such cases, but Eunice Stopfel said that about 20 percent of the cases one encounters do not respond either partially or completely. Do not expect miracles, though some do happen. And when there are instances that compression massage does not help, do not be discouraged.

Sometimes during the session there is an instant reaction: The feet and hands perspire so that they are practically wet and the person says that the whole body perspires. It is a purificatory response of the glands.

In one case a woman who came had severe bursitis and also marital problems — she was almost on the verge of divorce. After a few sessions her bursitis was gone and because she became calmer and more open-minded her marital problems disappeared. She told me "You saved my marriage — I wish I could take you home with me — it would make the whole family happy."

KARIN SCHUTT

Massage for Body & Soul

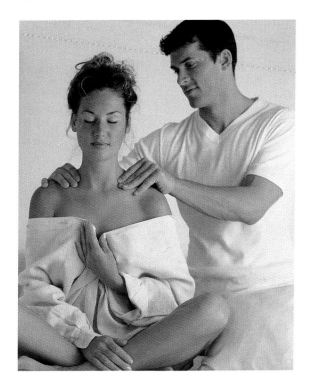

Sterling Publishing Co., Inc.
New York

Contents

Library of Congress Cataloging-in-Publication Data
Schutt, Karin.
    [Massagen. English]
    Massage for body & soul / Karin Schutt.
        p. cm.
    ISBN 0-8069-2037-8
    1. Massage. 2. Relaxation. 3. Stress management.
    4. Self-care. Health. I. Title. II. Title: Massage for
    body and soul.
RA780.5.S3813 1999
615.8'22—dc21   99–36725
                                              CIP

10 9 8 7 6 5 4 3 2 1

Published by Sterling Publishing Company, Inc.
387 Park Avenue South, New York, N.Y. 10016
Originally published and © 1997 by Gräfe and Unzer Verlag
GmbH, München, under the title *Massagen*
English translation © 1999 by Sterling Publishing Co., Inc.
Distributed in Canada by Sterling Publishing
c/o Canadian Manda Group, One Atlantic Avenue, Suite 105
Toronto, Ontario, Canada M6K 3E7
Distributed in Great Britain and Europe by Cassell PLC
Wellington House, 125 Strand, London WC2R 0BB, England
Distributed in Australia by Capricorn Link (Australia) Pty Ltd.
P.O. Box 6651, Baulkham Hills, Business Centre, NSW
2153, Australia
Printed in Hong Kong
All rights reserved

Sterling ISBN 0-8069-2037-8

An Important Note

Massages can help with many problems, but they cannot perform miracles. Sometimes, with certain diseases, a massage can even cause the symptoms to worsen or make the disease become more acute. Therefore, before you try to treat medical problems with massage, consult your doctor to find out if there are any medical reasons why massage may be unadvised. Also, please note the contraindications listed on page 68.

Self-massages, as they are introduced in this book, are obviously not as effective as receiving a massage from a trained massage therapist. Nevertheless, it is important to perform the massages correctly, because even "simple" massages can cause undesirable effects if they are administered the wrong way. The massages that appear in this book will not cause any problems even for beginners, as long as they adhere to the proper grip techniques (starting on page 27) and follow the instructions for the specific massages step by step.

Preface

Have you ever looked at your hands and thought about all the things that you have accomplished with them? According to the Greek philosopher Aristotle, our hands are the "best of all the tools." We can transform more than just our thoughts and feelings. With our hands, we can practice an art that is invaluable for our health. Massage, the art of stroking, kneading, and rubbing, is an ancient healing method whose therapeutic value is truly "in our own hands."

The hands are a tool whose touch can produce positive effects for us on many different levels. The hands can bring the body to a point from which it can start healing itself. They caress the soul and make us feel good, because we often don't need much more than being touched and held, and they relax us and set our spirits free. Massage is also a form of communication—a language without words—that brings us close together, connects us, and makes us more familiar with each other.

This book is an introduction to the versatile possibilities of using this all-encompassing healing method, and will show you how you can use massage in your everyday life as a source of beauty and health. You will find many helpful hints on how to give yourself and your partner simple, head-to-toe massages for relaxation, healing, and refreshing the body in a natural way. Because massage not only affects the body but also the soul and the mental state (perhaps them even more so), a regular practice of massage can help you and your partner reach an inner balance and stability.

Massage is a healthy activity for the entire family, it has no age limits, and as long as it is applied properly, it also has no harmful side effects. Give it a try!

Karin Schutt

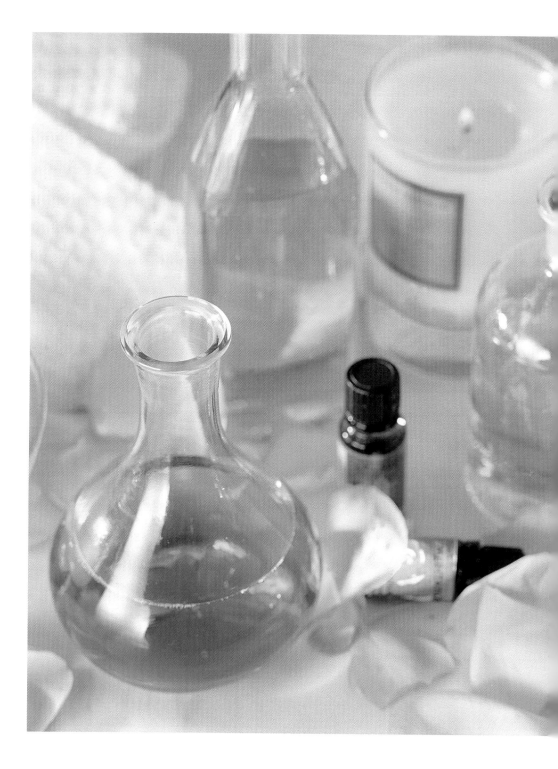

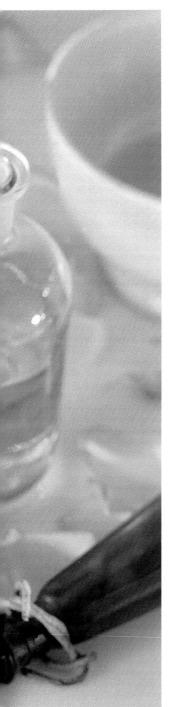

The Art of Massage

"Human beings beseech the gods for health, but they do not think of the fact that health lies in their own hands."
—Democritus (Greek philosopher, around 460 to 380 B.C.)

There is almost nothing that feels as good as getting a loving massage from a knowledgeable pair of hands with some scented oil. Various ancient cultures already knew of the healing power that lies in touch. Healing by hands is as old as the human race. Today, massage is scientifically recognized as a therapy that alleviates pain, heals, and improves general well-being.

In the pages that follow, you will learn about all the important effects and applications of massage as well as about oils and other accessories.

Knowledge of Healing Hands

When we greet each other, we shake hands; when we console children, we stroke their hair; when we want to express our love to someone, we gently caress that person. Through touch, we dissolve the boundaries of "I" and "you" and create a connection that goes far beyond the kinds of contact and understanding that can be expressed in words.

Touch is an elixir of life that all of us need in order to stay healthy physically, mentally, and spiritually. The hands play the most important role in touching, because they are sensory organs, information carriers, and transmitters of energetic powers all at the same time.

As soon as you touch your body or someone else's body with your fingertips and the palms of your hands, you receive information about the physical condition through the tactile sensation. The stimulation of touch releases healing physical reactions. The hands convey our intentions. Through them, we can send healing energy and create highly sensual pleasures. Massage is basically all this and even more.

The Healing Touch of Massage

All of us use massage instinctively. When a certain part of the body hurts, we lay our hands on it immediately and try to reduce the pain by applying circular motions to the sore area. When people are tense, it is often enough to simply lay your hand on them to help them relax.

These effects are also confirmed scientifically. When the skin is touched by other skin, it causes changes on both a physical and an emotional level. A loving touch can release certain hormones that are responsible for our well-being and feeling of happiness; at the same time, the nervous system receives impulses that have a relaxing effect on overtaxed nerves.

A strong impact on body and soul

By applying the healing touch of massage, we target those changes that can create balance in the organism as well as influence mood, ease pain, and release physical and emotional tensions (page 14).

Using Your Own Hands

Massage is a special kind of touch, a sort of "a dance on the skin," that is administered by a pair of trained hands with a lot of feeling in the fingertips. Every massage session turns into a relaxing experience when touch, technique, and rhythm all come together in the consciousness of the masseur.

■ In order to be able to apply this healing touch to yourself or another person, you will first need to understand a few basic ideas, which will be presented to you in the following sections. All the rest will develop by itself over time through regular applications of the self-massage and partner-massage exercises that are introduced in this book. If you wish to get further information, you could attend a course.

Precondition for treatment

Most adult education centers offer massage courses where you can learn the basics and practice the techniques.

Massage in Daily Life—a Tool for Healing and Pleasure

Massage is an excellent tool for increasing your own and your partner's sense of well-being. Especially in daily life—after a stressful week or from time to time, if possible, at the workplace—a relaxing massage can help you reduce your stress and charge your batteries with new energy.

Furthermore, the positive and relaxing effects of massage are as beneficial for babies and children as they are for adults.

Massage as a healing remedy

● Massage is a healing art whose targeted touch is not limited to the part of the body that receives the massage but affects the entire organism. Many everyday problems can be resolved and healed in this way (page 66).

For mental
balance
● Massage is a natural relaxant and stimulant for body, mind, and soul, because it creates balance physically, mentally, and spiritually (page 38).

● Regular massages are beautifiers, giving one a glowing look and a relaxed facial expression. The blood circulation in the skin is improved, lymphatic swelling in the face goes down, and wrinkles that are caused by tension become smooth (pages 22 and 52). For beauty

● Regular connective tissue massages of problem areas, such as the stomach, buttocks, and thighs, are not only soothing but also have a preventive effect as they stimulate the blood circulation of the skin and improve the condition of the connective tissue (page 54).

In sports
● Regular massages can be very effective as a fitness remedy. They make the muscles more elastic and help keep the joints feeling smooth. Applying massage before and after participating in sports reduces the danger of injury and contributes to the speedy regeneration of tired muscles (page 56).

● A partner massage can be one of sensual pleasure, awakening desire and leading to erotic adventures. A loving touch, trustworthy devotion, and the willingness to concentrate on the other person create the kind of intimacy that doesn't usually occur in such a natural and uninhibited way in daily life. Besides that, through massage, partners get the chance to become more familiar with each other's bodies and reactions—this is something that will be beneficial for and deepen every relationship. For sensual
experiences

Gentle Therapy with Powerful Results

Regardless of which massage method you use on yourself or your partner, the effect will always be intense and all-encompassing. After all, the skin is our largest organ. Not only does it protect the body, regulate temperature, and have a bearing on the immune system, but it also has another special purpose: about five million sensory cells in the skin are simply waiting to receive even the slightest stimulation, which they then pass on to a countless number of nerves.

The skin—
our largest
organ

A Stimulant for Self-Healing Powers

As soon as your hands touch skin, an immediate stimulation is set in motion. This is perceived by the smallest sensory areas (receptors), and the information is passed on to the brain (page 15). A soft touch generally has a relaxing effect, whereas a strong touch usually activates. Therefore, it can be said of massage therapy that outer stimulants bring about different physical reactions.

Massage leads to balance.

The purpose of an "activating therapy" is to remove a certain imbalance in the body, to restore balance to the organism, or to stimulate the body's own ability to heal. In order for any of these effects to take place, a true shift in the body needs to occur. Usually, the body is capable of balancing itself by turning on an "inner switch." But if the organism cannot conduct this process by itself, it may need some assistance from the outside. This assistance can come from a stimulating way of relaxing impulses.

Helpful Impulses

In massage therapy, balancing impulses are administered in various ways. The touch itself, which comes first, already makes you feel good and is a very effective stimulant. The stimulation stems from the pressure that is applied by the hands, the warmth that results from it, and the choice of various grip techniques that intensify the effect (page 27).

Stimulation through various measures

All of the balancing impulses release the self-healing potential of the organism and help it to put into effect its own mechanism of self-regulation. This is how, for example, tension can turn into relaxation, and constant stress into a general state of calm and recovery.

Nature Leaves Its Mark

The methods of massage therapy that you will find in this book are classified as largely physical therapies. The term "physical therapy" is derived from the Greek word *physis*, which means "nature."

The traditions of some methods of physical therapy go back thousands of years. These kinds of therapy use techniques that come almost exclusively from nature. Examples of natural healing agents are cold and hot temperatures and certain herbs. In the case of massage therapy, the hands are the primary natural agents that help to ease various problems.

Effective Healing on Every Level

An important form of medical treatment

Massage is one of the most important methods of medical treatment there is; it is extremely successful, and its efficacy has been proven medically. Stroking, kneading, and rubbing are forms of therapy that are recognized by conventional medicine and are prescribed either by themselves or in conjunction with other treatments. Trained massage therapists and physiotherapists often work together with medical practitioners at health spas and hospitals. Many practitioners of natural medicine receive additional training in massage therapy.

In Germany, for example, health insurance plans usually cover massage therapy as long as it is prescribed by a doctor. If you choose to get a massage from a healing practitioner, you would have to pay for it out of your own pocket. The same holds true for massage therapy that is administered by trained professionals when you request it "only" for relaxation.

What follows is an introduction to the various factors that in conjunction produce the healing effects of massage; all of these factors have been proven through medical research.

Relief for Body and Soul

The psycho-sedative effect

If you have ever experienced the pleasure of a good massage, you are aware of its positive effects. You can breathe deeply and heave a sigh of relief, for your tension and nervousness have abated and you can truly let go of inner burdens. You might even fall asleep during the massage—a sign of the deepest physical, mental, and spiritual relaxation. After the massage, your body feels light and warm. The calming and relaxing effect, which is also called the *psycho-sedative effect,* is one of the most pleasurable and beneficial results of the healing touch.

Stimulation for the Circulatory System

Massage increases the rate of local blood circulation by up to five times, both in the superficial and the deep layers of the tissue. This increased blood supply gives the cells plenty of oxygen and important nutrients. At the same time, the lymph system (page 22) is also stimulated, so that accumulated waste products and poisons can be filtered better and transported out of the body.

The medical term for the stimulation of blood circulation and lymph circulation is the *vascular effect*. Well-functioning circulation and a well-functioning lymph system are the preconditions for a well-functioning immune system.

The vascular effect

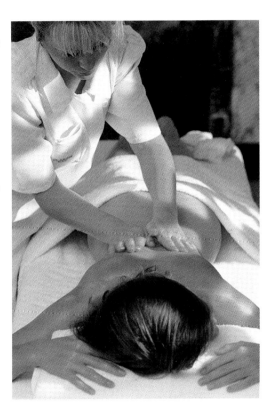

Recovery for Overtaxed Nerves

The balancing effect of massage on the nervous system, also known as the *neural effect*, is produced primarily by the warmth of the hands, the pressure applied by well-trained hands, and the stimulating touch.

The skin functions here as a transmitter of healing energy due to the innumerable nerve endings (receptors) that pass through it. These nerve endings receive stimulation constantly and pass it on through the nerves to the brain. Once the impulses reach the brain, which is our most important control and nerve center, they are processed and passed on to other parts of the body.

The neural effect

A form of therapy that is not only healing but can also be pleasurable

The various massage techniques can either stimulate or calm these nerve endings. As a result, tense nerves, which have become strained through stress, can rest and switch back to their normal functioning.

Harmonizing the Functions of the Organs

Massage even has a positive effect on the functioning of the body's internal organs. This effect, called the *segmental effect*, has to do with the connection between the internal organs and certain areas of the skin, and with the reflexive (automatic) reactions of the organs. Therefore, by massaging certain areas of the skin surface directly, we can exert an influence on the disturbances of specific organs, such as the kidneys, the liver, and the heart. The healing effects of foot reflexology and of connective tissue massage (pages 20–21) are based on this principle.

The segmental effect

Relaxation for Tense Muscles

Massage regulates the tension of the muscles. Tense muscles will relax, and flabby muscles will be toned. The purpose is to achieve a normal muscle tone. However, massage cannot be used as an indirect power-training method, because tight muscles can only develop through continuous muscular work (athletes who train on a regular basis can feel and see on their own bodies how their muscles get tighter and stronger).

The toning effect

The *toning effect* is created because muscles become more elastic and stretchable through the increased blood circulation caused by massage. This in turn reduces susceptibility to injuries, which is why it makes sense to get a massage before participating in sports. Massage also helps tired and exhausted muscles to recover more quickly.

Easing Pain

We often feel severe pain when our muscles are extremely tense. Regular and well-measured massage can be of assistance in such cases, because certain painful massage grips will overlap the existing pain (but not when the pain is caused by an infection or an injury!). The nerves send a new pain impulse to the brain that is stronger than the original pain signal and therefore overlaps it. This occurrence is referred to medically as the phenomenon of *override*, because a strong stimulation cancels out the effect of the weaker one.

The phenomenon of override

As the pain diminishes, muscular tension disappears along with it. This has a positive influence on blood circulation and therefore also on the blood supply to the tissue. In addition, the stimulation of touch sends a signal to the brain to activate the production of certain hormones. The brain produces, among other things, an increased quantity of endorphins, the body's natural painkillers, and, according to recent medical research, also the hormone oxytocin, which clearly calms stress reactions and has a pain-reducing effect as well.

The hormonal effect

An Ancient Natural Healing Method

Knowledge of healing hands is as old as humankind. Before you become engaged with the various kinds of massage and the different massage techniques, take some time to explore the history of this ancient healing method in order to understand its origins and its development up to now.

The History of Massage

We have proof that healing with massage goes back more than 5,000 years. In the teachings of the Ayurveda, which is an ancient Indian treatise on longevity and healthy living, massage is mentioned as a form of therapy that stimulates the self-healing powers within us, induces deep relaxation, and leads to the detoxification of the body. Also, in Chinese medicine, there is a long tradition of massage being used as a method of treating and preventing diseases. Acupressure is one of the Chinese forms of massage that is known in the West. Acupressure and Ayurvedic massage methods are two of the oldest massage therapies in the world.

The oldest methods originated in Asia.

A look at pre-Christian Roman and Greek history shows that massage was applied in the ancient world before and after athletic competitions, during recuperation from an illness, after bathing, and especially as a form of therapy for physical and emotional problems, such as digestive disorders, shortness of breath, and melancholy.

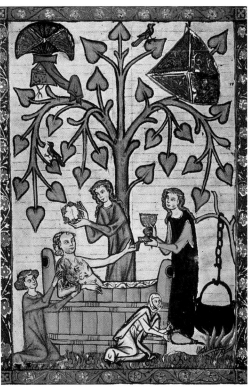

The Greek physician Hippocrates (approximately 460 to 375 B.C.), who is regarded as "the father of Western medicine," considered rubbing to be an art that every doctor had to possess. Later, it was the Greek physician Galen (approximately A.D. 129 to 199) who wrote about, among other things, specific massage techniques and their applications. However, as Christianity spread, touching became an object of general disapproval. For this reason, the ancient knowledge of the art of kneading was nearly forgotten. Since Christianity, the first written accounts of the application of massage are from the sixteenth century. The French doctor Ambroise Paré (1510 to 1590) developed a form of massage that he used particularly to support the healing processes.

The Greco-Roman tradition

Bathing was a favorite activity during the times of courtly love. Massage, on the other hand, was almost forgotten during the Middle Ages.

In the nineteenth century, the Swedish physiotherapist Per Henrik Ling and the Dutch doctor J. Georg Mezger finally helped the art of massage regain its former reputation. By the end of the nineteenth century, classical massage, which is based on the Greco-Roman massage tradition, became an essential aspect of medical treatments due to its pervasive success in therapy.

Rediscovery and establishment

After that, the techniques of classical massage were improved and made more sophisticated, and their results were backed up by scientific research. In addition to classical massage, there are various other forms of massage used today that either come from Asia (such as acupressure or Shiatsu) or were developed from the experience and recognition of Western doctors and massage therapists (such as connective tissue massage and foot reflexology).

Various Methods

In the following section, I would like to introduce you to five different methods of massage, all of which are recognized medically. These five massage methods will be combined in the various treatment concepts that you will encounter later in the book. For a short overview of other forms of massage, turn to page 24.

Classical Massage

The basis for most other methods

Many massage methods stem from the practice of "classical," or "Swedish," massage; its grip techniques—stroking, kneading, and rubbing—form the basis of the majority of massage methods. Detailed instructions for the application of these techniques begin on page 27. Classical massage serves one general purpose: it normalizes the tone of the skin and the muscles, while stimulating the circulation of the blood and the lymph.

In therapeutic practice, classical massage is used mainly to treat the following conditions:

Healing indications

- Rheumatic diseases
- Neurological disorders, such as paralysis
- Consequences of injuries and surgeries of the movement apparatus
- Internal diseases, such as heart problems, high blood pressure, shortness of breath, and bronchitis
- Psychosomatic problems, such as headaches, migraines, insomnia, digestive disorders, circulatory problems, exhaustion, and stress

Tense Muscles

Not only does the skin benefit from massage, but the muscles do as well. The muscles tense up when we move our bodies too little, the wrong way, or too much (professional athletes), when we remain more or less in the same position for hours at a time, when we are afraid, or when we are under constant inner stress.

Usually, muscles relax by themselves as soon as the problematic situation is over. Still, it often happens that a group of muscles or even just a few muscles create chronic tension in the muscular tissue, which over time ends up causing pain. A pain in the back or a stiff neck, for example, indicate that those parts of the body had pressure applied to them in the wrong way or were subjected to too much pressure over an extended period of time.

- Posture damages, such as curvature of the spine (scoliosis)
- Tension in the muscular area, such as cervical vertebra syndrome, dorsal vertebra syndrome, and lumbar vertebra syndrome
- Physical developmental impediments in children

Connective Tissue Massage

Connective tissue massage (CTM) is based on the expositions of the English neurologist Dr. Henry Head (1861 to 1940). He discovered that internal disorders and diseases can be seen on the skin, especially in the connective tissue. Certain skin surfaces are connected to internal organs by nerves and blood vessels. The stimulation of these areas of the skin (such as by massage) ends up affecting the internal organs in a balancing way and can even eliminate a disturbance completely. On the basis of this knowledge, German physiotherapist Elisabeth Dicke and physician Dr. Hede Teirich-Leube developed the therapeutic applications of connective tissue massage. On page 54, you will find a few grip techniques of CTM that can help you improve the appearance of skin with cellulite.

Effective for the connective tissue and the internal organs

Connective Tissue

Tight buttocks, smooth thighs, a flat stomach—connective tissue is responsible for them as well. Connective tissue is everywhere in the body; it literally holds us together by supporting the internal organs and connecting the bones. The delicate, light layers of tissue lie like a porous sponge under the outer layer of the skin. With their elastic fibers, the layers of connective tissue weave a thick net between the muscles, the fat tissue, and the skin.

Connective tissue leads the blood vessels, lymph passages, and nerves all the way to the surface of the skin, and it supplies them with nutrients and transports the waste products out of the system. The grip techniques of CTM—pulling and rolling—not only improve the supply of the connective tissue but also treat disorders of the internal organs that manifest themselves on the related skin surface as indentations, extensive dents, or swellings.

In therapeutic practice, connective tissue massage is used for the following:
- Blood circulation problems
- Lymphatic disorders
- Fluctuating blood pressure
- Sensation of freezing
- Functional disorders of internal organs and the area surrounding the organs, such as the

Healing indications

stomach and the intestinal system or the heart and the circulatory system
- Women's problems, such as disturbances related to menstruation or menopause
- Respiratory diseases, such as bronchitis or bronchial asthma

Foot Reflexology

"Show me your feet, and I will tell you about your health!" This was the motto of the British massage therapist Eunice D. Ingham. About sixty years ago, she developed a method of massage therapy based on the assumption that every organ area in the body relates to a certain area on the feet and hands, and that it can be influenced from that area. Such "reflex zones" are found on the soles of the feet and the palms of the hands as well as on the backs and the sides of the feet and the hands, below the ankles or the wrists. These zones reflect the situation of the organs. For instance, if a certain zone hurts when you massage it using the appropriate rubbing technique (page 29), this means that something is not quite right with the corresponding organ. In Germany, a debt of gratitude is owed to the massage therapist Hanne Marquardt for the increasing recognition and respect that reflexology now receives there from conventional medicine.

Influencing the organs through the feet and the hands

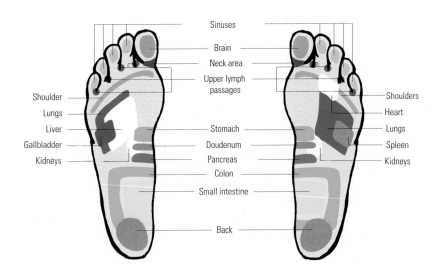

Some of the main reflex zones of the feet

In therapeutic practice, foot reflexology is used for the following:
- Functional disorders of specific organs or of systems that relate to specific organs
  - Migraines, headaches
  - Muscular cramps
  - Menstrual problems
  - Diseases of the respiratory apparatus
  - Stress, nervousness, sleeping disorders
  - Allergic reactions, such as hay fever

"Purification Plant" of the Body

The lymph system performs a very important function in the body, in that lymphatic fluids carry the accumulated waste products of the metabolic system. Especially large protein molecules that accumulate during infections find their way back into the blood through the lymph. Once they are in the blood, the body can get rid of them through the detoxifying organs (liver and kidneys).

If the lymph passages are damaged, or if the flow of the lymph is interrupted, the result is an accumulation of fluids in the tissue. The skin looks swollen, and any applied pressure to the swollen areas leaves a notch that takes some time to disappear. The assistance of mechanical hand pressure pushes the accumulated fluids in the tissue out of the body. In this way, the fluids are transported over the lymph nodes into the lymph passages and from there into the venous blood circulation.

Manual Lymphatic Drainage

Lymphatic drainage quickly removes metabolic waste products and overflowing lymph through the lymph passages. A hand massage ("manual" massage) in which circular motions and light pulling grips are applied along the lymph passages was developed in 1932 and later refined by the Danish physiotherapist Dr. Emil Vodder. An example of a case in which lymphatic drainage can be helpful is when the face and especially the area around the eyes appear swollen (page 52). Lymphatic drainage is therefore an important part of a professional cosmetic facial.

The effect of removing accumulated waste products and of detoxification

Manual lymphatic drainage is used as a therapy for the following:
- Removal of the lymph nodes, for the purpose of releasing

Healing indications

blockages of lymphatic fluids (edemas)
- Edemas that appear after accident-related injuries
- Diseases of the lymph vessels
- Vein-related problems—for example, to release the pressure from chronic "swollen legs"

Acupressure

Harmonizing the energy flow

Acupressure, or "finger-pressure massage," is, for Westerners, the most popular method of Chinese medicine. It is similar to acupuncture, in which the stimulation is produced with needles that are inserted into specific points. In acupressure, however, the healing stimulation is produced by the fingertips. Both methods are based on the theory of the meridians.

Acupressure acts on specific points of the meridians, influencing the Chi, our vital life energy.

The basic assumption is that there are energy passages, or "meridians," along the body through which our life energy, or "Chi," flows. When we are sick, the flow of life energy is interrupted. Targeted finger pressure on certain points along the meridians helps to remove an existing blockage of the energy flow, so that the life-giving Chi can flow again without interruption. The purpose of this Chinese fingertip massage is to influence the flow of the Chi by harmonizing it, relaxing it, or stimulating it.

Healing indications

Many massage therapists and healing practitioners use acupressure for the following:
- To activate life energy in various stages of fatigue, or as a relaxing treatment for nervousness
- To ease headaches, stomachaches, toothaches, or a sore throat
- To produce a balancing effect on the nervous system

Additional Special Forms of Massage

Over time, many forms of massage have developed in the West that combine traditional Eastern medicine with modern Western medicine or have entirely their own approach.

Pressure Point Massage, According to W. Penzel

This is also called meridian massage, because it is based on the theory of the meridians (page 23). The first step is conducted with the assistance of a massage stick, which is used along the meridians in either a slow or a fast motion to balance the energy flow. This is followed by stimulating the acupuncture points with a special vibrating appliance. Pressure point massage is especially useful for functional disorders, chronic pain, and prevention.

Based on the theory of the meridians

An-Mo Massage or Tui-Na Massage

Both of these forms of massage are part of traditional Chinese medicine. The massage is applied to the meridians with either strong or gentle grip techniques, such as tapping, pounding, kneading, pressing, stroking, or pulling. The blockages in the energy flow are released, creating a strong flow of energy. The obstructions can be triggered by numerous problems, including functional disorders of the internal organs, chronic pain, and diseases of the bones or the limbs.

Chinese massages for the release of energy blockages

Biodynamic Massage, According to Gerda Boyesen

"Healing the soul through the body" is the motto of this psychotherapeutic massage. It is based on the idea that the organism possesses the ability to influence our feelings and problems through muscular tension and chronic tension of the diaphragm. Targeted breathing exercises combined with specific massage techniques set a dynamic process in motion. In this process, patients get access to their subconscious.

Psycho- therapy through the body

Colon Massage

Chronic or acute digestive disorders, such as constipation, can be treated successfully with this special stomach massage.

Assistance for digestion

Craniosacral Work

Strengthening the immune system and self-healing powers

This form of therapy is concerned with the rhythm of the brain fluids and the fluids of the spinal chord that pulse within the skull, or the cranium, and along the spine, all the way to the sacrum. The disruption of the rhythm of this movement has a negative effect on our overall physical and mental well-being. By means of a delicate touch, craniosacral massage restores the healthy and regular craniosacral rhythm, in order to stimulate the body's immune system and set the healing process in motion. This therapy has proven to be effective in cases of muscle spasms, headaches, migraines, allergies, and ringing in the ears.

Periosteum Massage

The periosteum (the membrane of connective tissue that closely enfolds all bones except at the surfaces of joints) is a very sensitive organ due to the numerous nerves and blood vessels it contains. This is why periosteum massage was developed by two German doctors as a method of relieving pain. Some kinds of pain (but not pain caused by infections or injuries) can be relieved by a specific form of pressure that is applied to certain points on the bones. The original pain from the inside is thus eliminated by the pain from the outside, which is caused by the applied pressure of the fingers.

Effective against pain

Polarity Massage, According to Dr. Rudolph Stone

Release of energy blockages

This form of massage is based on the natural law according to which the human body is divided by a pattern of electromagnetic polarity, just as everything else in nature is. The top of the body (the head) and the right half of the body are positively charged, whereas the left half of the body and the feet are negatively charged. By means of specific massage, touch, and stretching techniques, this form of massage releases and balances the existing energy blockages in the magnetic field of the body.

Rolfing, According to Ida Rolf

Rolfing improves posture by shortening or stretching the muscles, in order to return them to their original tone. This effect is achieved by means of applying rough, strong pressure and specific

Eases tension

hand grips. Because muscular tension is often a result of mental tension, the relief of those muscles can lead to an increasing awareness of one's emotional problems, which is often experienced during a rolfing session. Rolfing is therefore often combined with psychotherapy.

Shiatsu

The Japanese version of acupressure

Shiatsu ("shi" means finger, and "atsu" means pressure) is the Japanese version of Chinese finger-pressure massage, or acupressure, described on page 23. Shiatsu is also based on the idea that energy channels, or meridians, are in the body and that life energy (Chi) flows through them. In the event of an illness, the blocked Chi can be set into motion by the application of specific hand grips along the meridians.

Thai Massage

The Indian version

This form of massage originated in India. Similar to Shiatsu and acupressure, Thai massage is based on the idea that certain channels of life energy (in this case, prana) run through the body. Delicate hand grips along these energy channels cause the prana to resume its flow, and this in turn can relieve pain and heal disorders.

Underwater Massage

This massage entails water pressure coming out of a water hose. It is conducted with warm water, at temperatures ranging from 93 to 100 degrees F (34 to 38 degrees C). It has a very relaxing effect and stimulates the blood circulation of the skin. Underwater massage is generally used after operations and for pulled ligaments and bruises.

Relaxation when you have pain

Yin and Yang Massages

Balance between active and passive energy

This method is based on the Chinese system of two complementary opposites: yin—an emotional, passive, and soothing energy—and yang—an active, dynamic force. Ideally, these two different forces should be in harmony in every human being, but in reality, one of them usually has the upper hand. This form of massage balances out the excess yin or yang energies, in order to provide health for both body and soul. The yin massage is very relaxing, whereas the yang massage is a real energizer.

Basic Course in Massage

Before you start giving massages, it is important to familiarize yourself with the basics of massage therapy. This way, your massages will become a positive and recovering experience for each of your massage partners and for yourself.

Massage itself is very easy to learn, but there are other important aspects to it that are helpful to understand. It is recommended that you read the introductions to the different grip techniques and the tips regarding preparation and practice before you start the exercises. This way, your massages will not only improve your partners' general well-being and cause them to relax, but you will also avoid feeling insecure and making mistakes during massages.

A good atmosphere is important, as it increases the effectiveness of the massage. A pleasant smell creates a comfortable, pleasing atmosphere.

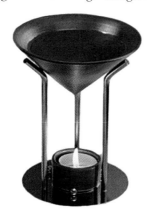

Grip Techniques

In this section, you will learn the basic grip techniques of classical massage. When you finish reading this section, it is advised to try the hand grips on yourself or on a partner before you go on to offer someone a full massage. This will help you acquire a sense for this special form of touch. Besides that, you will learn how the skin and the muscles feel and how to apply soft and strong grips without releasing uncomfortable physical sensations.

Practice increases self-confidence.

Stroking (Gentle Massage)

Each of the massages described in the following chapters starts with gentle stroking, in order to:

- Establish the first contact with the skin
- Get yourself and your partner in the mood for a massage
- Spread the massage oil on the skin

Gentle stroking at the beginning of every massage

• Prepare the area for more intensive treatment

Gentle strokes achieve these effects:

Effects
• Light stimulation of blood circulation and lymph circulation in the treated area
• Release of surface tension
• Enhancement of the general process of relaxation

Strong, deep stroking
After applying the initial gentle strokes and other grip techniques that establish contact, you can start using deeper strokes with stronger pressure, in order to:
• Produce stronger blood circulation and lymph flow

Effects
• Acquire a first impression of the state of the muscles (soft or hard)
• Improve the general tension of the muscles (tone)
• Stimulate your partner's breathing (deeper breathing)
• Effect your partner's emotional release (worries are stroked away, stress is massaged out, and thinking quiets down)

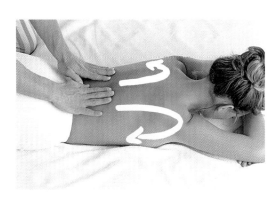

➤ Create upward strokes with both palms of the hands. By slightly bending the upper body, you apply gentle, even pressure. For deeper strokes, apply more pressure on the base of the palms. Then slide your hands back to the beginning position without applying any pressure.

Stroking: Gentle or with pressure, slide your hands flat over the skin.

Kneading

Stroking is followed by the more intensive grip technique of kneading, which has the following effects:
• It relieves general muscular tension and makes the hard muscles gradually become softer and more flexible.
• It works through both the underlying layer of fat as well as the muscle fiber.
• The waste products that accumulate in the veins and in

Effects

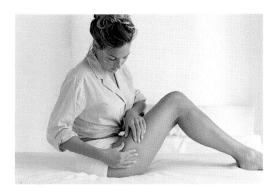
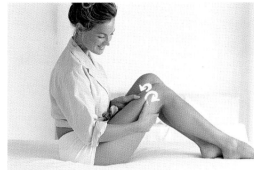

the lymph passages can be transported out of the body quickly due to the strong stimulation of the blood circulation.

➤ Take a large area of the skin between the tips of your fingers, and manipulate it as if you were kneading bread dough: press, push, and roll this meaty muscle tissue.

Rubbing (Friction)

For rubbing, you need only one thing: sensitivity in your fingertips. Try it as often as possible on yourself or on a partner. You will see how effective this grip technique is. Use it to:

• Feel and resolve even the slightest muscle hardening
• Relieve muscle pain
• Support the discharge of waste products

➤ Apply pressure to the front of the thumbs, and rub the skin in small circular motions, without losing contact with the skin. For greater intensity, open the circles and rub in spirals. Switch rhythmically between the circular and spiral motions.

Swinging (Vibrations)

An intensive treatment is usually followed by relaxing and calming hand grips. These can be either stroking or other grip techniques, such as swinging, that get the skin moving. By doing so, you achieve the following effects:
• Slight stimulation of the entire nervous system
• Relaxation of the muscles that have previously received intensive treatment
• Deepened breath

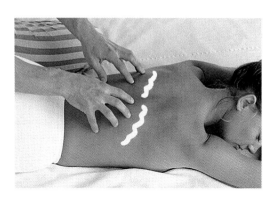

▶ Set all your fingertips on the skin, shake them slightly forward and backward, while moving the hands away from each other. These wavy motions are known as "swinging."

Practice Tips

While practicing the various grips, it's important to pay attention to the following pointers:
- Always touch the body of your partner with both hands, even if you are only massaging with one hand. The constant physical contact will give your partner a feeling of security.

- When you change your position or the grip technique, you should leave at least one hand on your partner's body so that you don't break the continuity of the contact.
- It is essential for the relaxation that you want to achieve to keep a flowing rhythm to the massage. Therefore, avoid any jerky, abrupt motions, especially when you change from one grip technique to another.

- Try to keep this basic rule of massage in mind: certain grip techniques are administered in the same direction as that of the blood flow and the lymph flow, toward the heart and the center of the body. For example, when you massage the arms of your partner, you should generally start with the hands and gradually move upward toward the shoulders (toward the heart). The same holds true for the legs: generally stroke from the feet upward toward the hips.

The Right Grip—Appropriate for the Condition

The choice of the right massage technique should be made according to the principle of balance. This means that:
- If your partner is in a general state of nervousness, you should choose the calming grips, such as stroking and light muscle vibrations.
- If your partner is in a general state of exhaustion and fatigue, after establishing the initial contact you can start with energizing and stimulating grip techniques.

Massage Preparation

There are many aspects of massage that you should pay attention to if you want to achieve an optimal effect.

Massage Oils Are Essential

Essential as a lubricant

Massage oils not only feel pleasant on the skin, but they are also essential for massage. They make it possible for the hands to slide over the skin and relieve the tense areas in an effortless and smooth way.

➤ When it comes to body oils, it's helpful to be aware of the following:

Tips for use

• Warm oils feel especially good on the skin. Therefore, it is always a good idea to slowly warm up a small amount of massage oil in hot water before you begin a massage.
• The advice is, less is always more, as far as oils are concerned. The skin doesn't need much of this substance in order to become smooth and pliable. If you pour on too much massage oil, simply absorb it with a soft napkin or a paper towel.
• First pour the oil into your (warm) hands, rub your hands

Aromatic Oils

You can either buy prepared massage oils (at the drugstore or the health food store) or simply use vegetable oils, such as almond oil, jojoba oil, or aloe vera oil.

• When you mix essential oils (which can also be purchased at drugstores and health food stores) with a vegetable oil, it is a pleasant experience for the skin and the senses. The healing and aromatic components of the oil affect the skin and the sense of smell, enhancing the overall positive effect of the massage.
• With the descriptions of the different massages, you will find more tips on pleasant-smelling and healing massage oils.
• It is very important to use high-quality oils. Therefore, buy only 100 percent pure essential oils and plant oils from the first cold pressing, all of which should be, if possible, certified as organic products.

➤ When you want to mix it yourself: Take 50 ml (a little less than 4 tablespoons) of a plant oil, add a total of 10 to 20 drops of an essential oil (with strong oils, such as rose or cedar, 1 to 2 drops is enough!), and shake the bottle before use. The aroma will take a week or two to "round up."

The mixture can hold as long as the date indicated for its individual components. If the oil is "overdue," it will smell bad.

together a little, and then spread the oil evenly over your partner's skin.

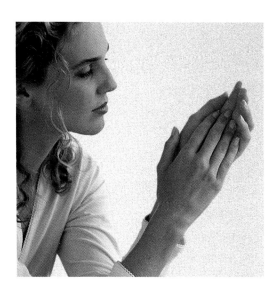

A formula with balancing and relaxing effects for an aromatic oil lamp:
3 drops of geranium oil
1 drop of rose oil
1 drop of cedar oil
First put some water in the cup of the aroma lamp, and then add the ethereal oils.

Formula for an aromatic oil lamp

Before Using Your Hands

Before you give a massage, it's important to look at your hands and check the following: Do you have long fingernails, are your hands cold, or are you wearing rings, a watch, or a bracelet? All this will not only interfere with the pleasant, relaxing effect of the massage but can even lead to disagreeable or dangerous consequences (long fingernails or jewelry, for example, can cause injuries!).

Essential preparation

> This is what you need to do to avoid having cold hands: take a warm hand bath (approximately two minutes in warm water, at 95 to 100 degrees F, or 35 to 38 degrees C), and then dry your hands forcefully. After that, rub your hands against each other as long as it takes for them to radiate a pleasant warmth.

Remedy for cold hands

Before a massage, dedicate yourself to taking care of your hands.

The Senses Also Need Relaxation

Turn your massage room into a haven of tranquillity and security; anything that caresses the senses will improve your sense of well-being. The better the atmosphere, the easier it will be to switch off and relax. Therefore, try to provide the following conditions:
• Your massage room should be a comfortable temperature.
• It's important not to be disturbed during the massage (turn off the doorbell, turn on the answering machine, and so forth).
• Put on some quiet, relaxing music, light some candles, and take advantage of pleasant aromas to soothe the senses.

Create an oasis of relaxation.

Locating Tenseness

Usually, we are aware of our most problematic areas, the ones in which muscular tension always reappears. For example, the musculature in the back and the neck often tends to tense up, harden, or cramp. During the massage, you can also track down the typical characteristics of these tense areas.

What Do the Muscles Feel Like?

Soft and elastic, or hard and tight?

You will realize that a relaxed muscle feels relatively soft and elastic. You can raise it easily, rub it with your fingertips, or forcefully knead through it. However, if you feel small knots in the muscular tissue or if you feel a hard, tight cord, there is a local cramp or a general cramp of an entire group of muscles.

Does the Massage Hurt?

A cramped, hardened muscle hurts when it is being massaged. A piercing or muffled pain indicates that the muscles in a given area are very tight.

Important: Massaging bones becomes unpleasant. You should therefore pay attention not to work on bony areas, such as the spine.

Never massage the bones!

How Does the Skin React?

The skin also gives you some important hints during the massage. Its signals are related to the strength of the massage. When you massage soft and relaxed muscles, the skin reacts with a slight reddening. However, if you stroke, rub, or knead a cramped muscle, the skin will become fire-red to dark red.

Slight or intense reddening

Treating Cramps

Muscle pain can be alleviated if you first start with the gentle grip techniques, such as stroking and swinging. Advance slowly to the more intensive grip techniques, like kneading and rubbing.

Adjust your applied pressure to your partner's level of pain sensitivity. The more sensitive you are in this process, the more relaxed your partner will be. Afterward, follow up with the calming grips. You can repeat this entire process three times. Ask your partner during the process to breathe deeply and not to hold his or her breath.

The Right Position

It is of utmost importance when you are getting a massage to be lying or sitting down comfortably.

A Relaxing Way of Lying Down

It is uncomfortable to lie on a surface that is too hard, too soft, or uneven. Appropriate massage surfaces are a mattress that is not too soft, a large table with some padding, and a firm bed or sofa. You need to be able to approach the surface on which the massage takes place from all sides. If you intend to give massages on a regular basis, consider buying a special massage table.

The appropriate surface

A Relaxing Way of Sitting

Wear loose, comfortable clothing. Sit straight but relaxed on a chair, with your feet placed flat on the floor. If you give yourself a head massage, a comfortable way of sitting is to rest your elbows on a table. You will find further hints in the chapters describing specific forms of massage.

How You Can Really Get Comfortable

Sitting or lying down can be made more comfortable if you use pillows as well as neck rolls (made out of rolled-up towels). This also helps prevent the exertion of too much pressure on certain areas. In order to keep the body warm during the massage, it is helpful to use warm flannel sheets or wool blankets.

Using pillows, bed sheets, and blankets

Important: Warmth supports relaxation during a massage. The feet especially tend to cool down over the course of a massage. In this case, warm socks or a hot water bottle can be helpful.

Warmth is important.

Correct Posture When Giving a Massage

When you are giving a massage, you should also wear loose and comfortable clothing and keep a relaxed posture. If you apply the massage while sitting on your knees, it would be a good idea to put a pillow underneath them. In any case, be mindful of not swaying your back during the session. If possible, you should work while keeping your back straight. Massage therapy is less tiring from the standing position if you bend your knees slightly when applying pressure.

Staying as relaxed as possible

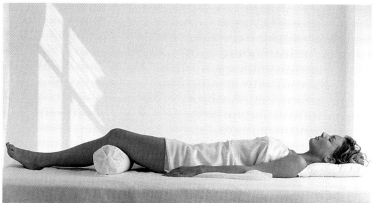

When lying on your back, it is helpful to have small pillows supporting the back, the hollow of the knees, and the neck.

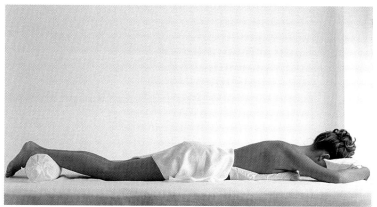

Lying on the stomach is made more comfortable by placing pillows under the forehead, the chest and stomach area, and the feet.

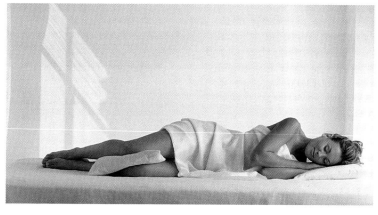

If you lie on your side, it is helpful to put pillows under your head and between your legs.

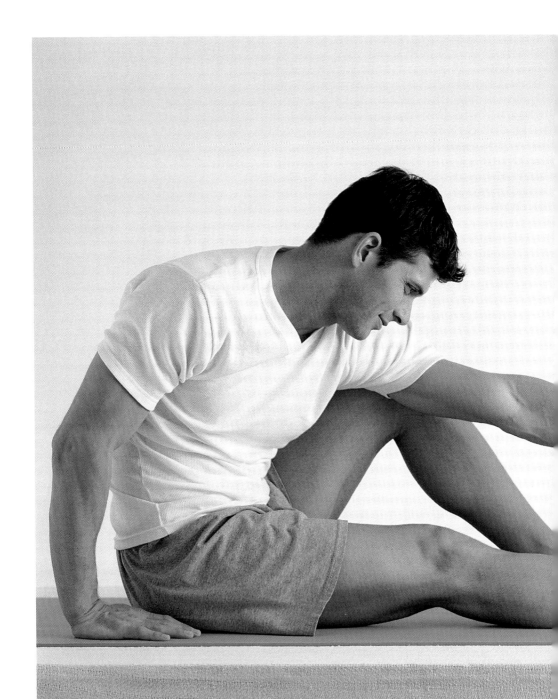

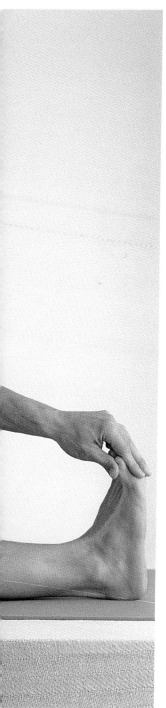

Fit and Beautiful through Massage

"A kind touch can promote energy, enjoyment of life, and self-awareness."
—Yehudi Menuhin (American violinist and conductor)

Massage is a positive experience on many different levels: it helps the body recover and regenerate itself, it caresses the soul, and it transmits a feeling of security and being cared for. In addition, it alleviates pain and prevents disorders "with a light hand." Whether you want to pamper yourself, your partner, or your child, massage can be a regular beautifier, relaxant, stimulator, fitness cure, or loving caress. But it needs to be approached the right way.

Caressing Body and Soul

Warm hands stroking the skin and kneading and rubbing the muscles: even though we only touch the surface of the body, we also touch the soul. Massages have a profound, all-encompassing effect.

Balance and energy
All the physical and emotional baggage that we bring with us to a massage session will be worked through, balanced out, and, when necessary, driven out of the body. This way, body and soul can recover, become refreshed, and accumulate new energies.

If you come to a massage session feeling exhausted and sad, for example, you will discover that after the massage your feelings will have changed drastically: streams of warmth will fill your body, and you will feel elastic and flexible; the emotional pain will have lessened or disappeared altogether, and you will feel light, exhilarated, and calm.

Important: Before you begin, please note the suggestions regarding massage preparation starting on page 31 and the lists of contraindications on page 68.

Anti-stress Massages

A gentle massage with scented oils, in a pleasant atmosphere, is like a short vacation. The nervous system can switch from its constant activity into a state of pleasurable relaxation. Deep breathing makes it easier to let go of thoughts and internal tensions. Body and soul can recover from the exhaustion of daily life.

Recovering, as if you took a short vacation

Relaxing Body Oils

Certain body oils have a relaxing effect, ease tension, and create balance—choose your favorite scent.

Take 50 ml (a little less than 4 tablespoons) of jojoba or sweet almond oil, and add:

2 drops of rose oil
6 drops of lavender oil
   or
6 drops of bergamot oil
2 drops of ylang-ylang oil
2 drops of Siamese benzoin oil
   or
7 drops of orange oil or grapefruit oil
1 drop of muscatel sage oil
2 drops of sandalwood oil

Ways Massages Are Effective

Relaxation when you are stressed out, worried, or scared

- At night, before you go to bed, ask your partner to give you a massage, or simply give yourself one. It will improve your ability to fall asleep and to sleep through the night.
- During the day, at work, it is helpful to give yourself a massage. It prevents stress and all its consequences, such as nervousness, poor concentration, and fatigue.
- Worries and fear can be lessened with a massage.

Partner Massage

One of the most pleasurable experiences we can have after a long day at work is a relaxing massage from our spouses or partners. The back massage is especially effective for deep relaxation of the entire body, because a large number of nerves and nerve fibers stem from the spine and tangle up in various other parts of the body.

Also helpful for children

Children can also be under pressure, so the following exercises are appropriate for massaging the backs of small children as well.

➤ See "Massage Preparation" starting on page 31.
Prepare the warm oil, and place it next to

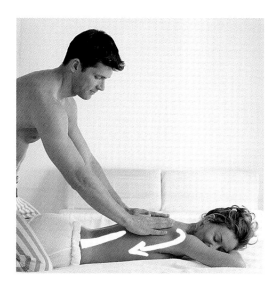

you. Your partner should be lying on his or her stomach, and you should cover your partner's legs to keep them warm. Stand or kneel down by your partner's side (if you are kneeling, place a pillow under your knees).

1 Spread some massage oil (approximately 1 teaspoon) between your warm hands.
- Lay your hands softly next to each other on the lower back, beneath the waist. Apply slight pressure on your hands by slightly bending your upper body.
- Slowly stroke the muscle fibers along the left and right sides of the spine, toward the base of the neck. Then stroke sideways, over the shoulders, to the sides of the back.

A balm for the soul: a gentle back massage. Starting with wide, outward, surface strokes always feels good.

From there, let your hands move without any applied pressure to the sides of the hips, and from there, with half a circle, inward toward the spine.
• You can repeat this upward stroke and soft upward slide as long as needed to spread the oil evenly (or at least six times).

2 Now lay only the base of your palms on the lower part of the back.
• Apply a slightly stronger pressure by bending your upper body, while slowly

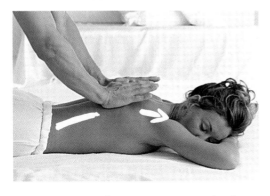

stroking your partner's back with the base of both your palms in an upward motion— not on the spine, but the muscles next to it!
• When you reach the neck, release the pressure; rest your hands on the shoulders, and then slide them down along the sides of the back.

• Repeat this deep stroking six times. Ask your partner to breathe in every time your hands slide up and to breathe out every time your hands slide down.

3 Lay your hands on your partner's lower back, about 4 in. (10 cm) away from each other.
• With some applied pressure, stroke in wide circular motions

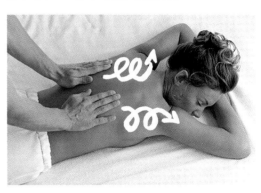

with both of your hands. Make slow, smooth, upward, rhythmical motions, following the contours of the body, and cover the sides as well.
• When you reach the neck, let your hands softly slide down.
• Repeat the circular outward strokes for a total of three times.

4 The following is a stroking grip technique that is ideal for the sides of the back:

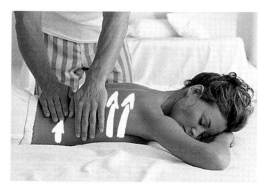

Stroking the sides

• Lay your hands opposite each other on one of your partner's hips. Pull your flat hands one after the other in a rhythmical fashion from the outside toward the inside, toward the spine, and slowly work your way up to the shoulders.
• Pulling the shoulders will create a very good sensation.
• After massaging the shoulders, let your hands slowly slide down.
• Repeat these pulling strokes at least three times.
• Then change your position, in order to massage the other side of the body.

Important: While changing your position, make sure always to leave one hand in contact with your partner's body (page 30).

5 To close the session, apply a relaxing and calming grip. This grip will help your partner calm down, and it will support the sensation of an inner connection between the upper and lower parts of the body.
• Lay one hand on the lower part of the spine, on the sacrum, and with the other hand softly hold your part-

Calming and connecting

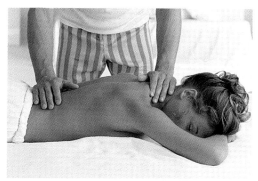

ner's neck. While doing this, try to compose yourself inwardly. Breathe in and out audibly several times, and ask your partner to do the same.
• After about a minute, slowly remove your hands; then cover your partner's back with a warm blanket, and allow him or her to relax for at least another ten minutes.

It is important to relax after a massage.

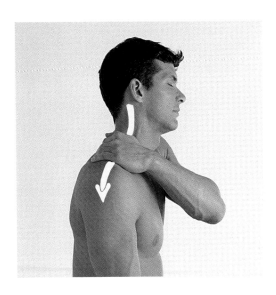

Self-Massage

We may not always have a partner available who can massage our stress away. But we can bring about relaxation ourselves by laying our own hands on our bodies. A shoulder massage and a neck massage can help smooth out and release the muscles that got tense as a result of stress.

➤ You can practice this kind of self-massage almost any time and any place: in the office, on the bus, or at home. The reason for this is that this massage doesn't require any preparation and you don't necessarily have to get undressed for it. So, sit down comfortably and begin.

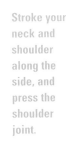

1 Put your right hand at your hairline above your left ear, and slowly stroke down along the left side of your neck toward the left shoulder joint.
• Press your shoulder joint firmly once, and then let your hand slide back.
• Repeat this stroke for a total of three times, before moving on to stroking the right side with the left hand.

Stroke your
neck and
shoulder
along the
side, and
press the
shoulder
joint.

2 Place both your hands around your neck, so that your fingertips meet at the back of your neck on your spine.

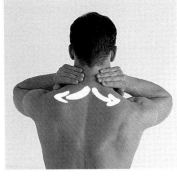

Stroking the
neck in har-
mony with
they rhythm
of the breath

• Close your eyes, and slowly push your hands with some applied pressure forward to the collarbone. Breathe out while pushing forward; breathe in while letting your hands slide back.
• Repeat this very relaxing stroke a total of five times.

3 Now lay your hands on your shoulders, so that your fingertips point backward toward the shoulder blades. Close your eyes.

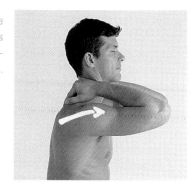

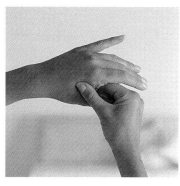

Apply rhythmic pressure to the point on the hand known as "dew fall."

- Apply pressure to the fingertips, and push them very slowly forward toward the collarbone.
- Once you reach the collarbone, let your fingertips softly slide backward.
- Repeat this stroke for a total of three times.

- Release the pressure for about two seconds, and then apply firm pressure again.
- Afterward, press the point on the back of the right hand with the left thumb.
Duration: One minute on each hand.

Acupressure—First Aid for Stress

Applying acupressure on the following points provides quick relaxation and brings about tranquillity:

1 Apply light pressure to the point on the back of the left hand (shown in photo) with the thumb of the right hand. Hold it for approximately ten seconds.

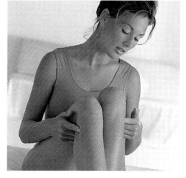

Apply constant pressure to the point below the knees known as "divine equanimity."

2 With both index fingers at the same time, apply light pressure to the points located about one hand width below each knee.
Duration: Up to five minutes.

Energizing Massages

Massage can also be a stimulant; its effects are similar to those produced by a cool shower.
• Quick and strong grips, applied with lively and aromatic massage oils, increase the energy level of body and soul, making fatigue and exhaustion disappear.
• An energizing massage has a reviving effect on the mental level as well. You will be able to think more clearly and your powers of concentration will improve—for example, before exams or important meetings. It also helps children concentrate better, such as when they do their homework.

Reviving Massage Oils

Certain massage oils will pep you up: they are refreshing and stimulating and improve concentration.
Take 50 ml (a little less than 4 tablespoons) of jojoba oil or sweet almond oil, and add:
6 drops of lime oil, lemon oil, or lemongrass oil • 3 drops of rosemary oil • 3 drops of cypress oil
or
2 drops of peppermint oil • 8 drops of grapefruit oil • 2 drops of hyssop oil
or
6 drops of petit-grain oil • 4 drops of silver fir oil • 2 drops of juniper oil

• Furthermore, an energizing massage supports recovery after a long illness.

Important: Because they have a stimulating effect, these massages should be avoided in the evening and at bedtime; they should only be administered when you still have plans for the day or wish to be especially alert.

Not before going to sleep!

Ten-Minute Partner Massage

If you want to awaken and pep up you partner, it's important for you yourself to be well rested and full of energy. The hand grips demand some talent and concentration.

The quick reviving massage fits into any schedule, no matter how packed it is. Because it doesn't require undressing, it can be done in the office or during breaks at various events.

Simple and easy to do any time

However, when you do the massage at home and use massage oil, it is recommended that your partner undress. For "Massage Preparation," see page 31.

➤ Your partner should sit up straight facing the back of the chair with his or her forearms supported by a small pillow. A bench can also be used.

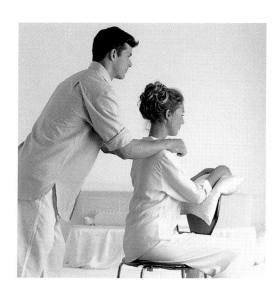

ly. Repeat these movements at least ten times.

3 Sit down or squat, and start massaging your partner's back with the palms of your hands. Make short, rapid motions along both sides of the spine, moving upward. Let your hands rest for a moment, pull them back slightly, and then quickly push them upward.

When you reach the shoulders, push down on them slightly.

First apply slight pressure on the shoulders . . .

1 Stand behind your partner, and rest your forearms against the muscles of his or her shoulders. Lean slightly forward, so that the weight of your body pushes down a little on your partner's shoulders. As you do this, your partner should exhale.
● Then reduce the pressure, and have your partner inhale.
● While your partner breathes out, support yourself with his or her shoulders.
● Repeat this three times in total.

. . . and then rub them back and forth.

2 Next, stroke both of your partner's shoulders with your forearms. Exerting slight pressure, move forward and backward fast and rhythmical-

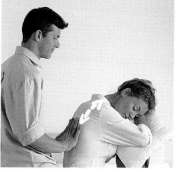

Rhythmically stroke both sides of the spine, moving upward.

Then stroke the shoulders in one flowing outward motion. Curve your hands over the upper arms, and allow them to slide back to the beginning position over the shoulders. Repeat this for a total of six times.

Kneading
the shoulder
musculature

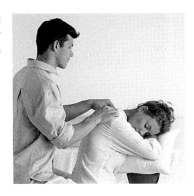

your body forward. Hold the pressure for a few seconds.

● Then move the thumbs about half an inch (1 centimeter) higher on the back, and in this fashion work your way up to the shoulders.

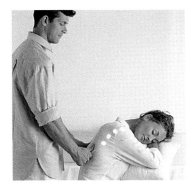

With the thumbs, apply pressure to both sides of the spine.

4 Knead the shoulder muscles on both sides of the neck, using both hands at the same time.

● Press, push, and drum on the muscles thoroughly, while applying force. In this way, work through the shoulder muscles and the muscles of the upper arms.

● Afterward, let your hands slide back to the starting position.

● Repeat the kneading massage for a total of three times.

5 Place the balls of your thumbs on your partner's lower back, to the left and to the right of the spine. You should start from a sitting or squatting position and then rise up to a standing position, as you work your way up the back.

● Apply pressure to the thumbs by slightly bending

● Then press the shoulder muscles half an inch by half an inch.

● Finally, let your hands slide back down, and start again with the muscles along the spine.

● Repeat the entire procedure for a total of three times.

6 Complete the energizing massage with the rhythmical strokes of the back described in Step 3.

A Quick Self-Massage

Stimulate the life force with acupressure

A stimulating point on the little finger increases blood circulation and wakes us up.
- Press this point (as an exception) with your (short) thumbnail.
Duration: Thirty seconds of pressure.

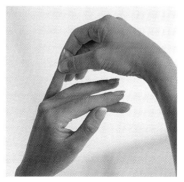

Press the point known as the "fast approaching wave."

Vibrant after Work, Relaxed for Sleep . . .

If you come home in the evening feeling tired but still have plans, you will find the following tips helpful in gaining a new serge of energy:

- The energizing massage and acupressure are both very useful.
- Stand next to an open window, and slowly breathe in through the nose and out through the mouth. Repeat this five times.
- If you have enough time, take a five-minute shower in which you switch from hot to cold water a couple of times. This will certainly wake you up.

After a busy day, if you encounter difficulties trying to switch off and fall asleep, try some of these suggestions:

- Sit down and relax for a couple of minutes, and then review the day in your mind.
- Treat yourself to the anti-stress-massage, described on page 42.
- Take a warm bath (98 to 100 degrees F, or 37 to 38 degrees C) in which you have added 5 drops of valerian oil. Bathing time should not exceed twenty minutes.
- While taking the bath, put on some quiet, relaxing music and let the day slowly wind down.

Beautiful from Head to Toe

Stress and a hectic lifestyle leave their marks: we look tired and tense, and the first signs of wrinkles start to appear on our faces. Treating yourself to a massage on a daily basis is like a beautifying treatment for body and soul.

With targeted hand grips and nurturing massage oils, you can do wonders for your internal and external well-being.

Massage as a Skin-Care Treatment

Almost no one has perfect skin. Whether your skin tends to look pale, is very dry and flaky, or has impurities, the stimulating effect of a massage and the grooming and nurturing benefits of massage oils will certainly help. The condition of your skin will eventually improve if the blood circulation in the skin is stimulated on a regular basis.

Effective for skin problems

• A full-body massage in the morning will make you fit for the day, and your skin will feel as soft as velvet, have good blood circulation, and receive all the nutrients that it needs.

• A facial massage will smooth out the wrinkles of sorrow and give you a relaxed appearance.

• If you have cellulite, a regular connective tissue massage will be helpful as it will clearly improve both the appearance and the feel of your skin.

For daily care or combating cellulite

Ayurvedic Oil Massage

The whole-body massage, which will soon be introduced to you, is part of the Indian Ayurveda (see page 17).

"Mature" Sesame Oil

According to the Ayurvedic tradition, sesame oil when used as a massage oil makes the skin smooth and slows down the aging process. But it is necessary to get hold of sesame oil of the highest quality. It has to be cold pressed, and it needs to be prepared to last for a long time without losing any of its ingredients that nourish the skin. High-quality sesame oil is available at health food stores and drugstores.

How the oil is prepared is important.

Warm up approximately100 ml (7 or 8 tablespoons) of sesame oil in a small pot to about 230 degrees F (110 degrees C). You can control the temperature by either using a thermometer or adding 2 drops of water to the warm oil. In the case of the latter, as soon as the oil reaches the right temperature, the drops of water will burst, making an audible sound. Now the oil is "mature" and ready to be used for massage. Allow the oil to cool down before applying it. If stored in a well-sealed glass bottle, this oil can be kept for up to six months.

Self-Massage from Head to Toe

➤ Perform this massage in the morning, even before you take a shower or a bath.

After you have done the massage, take a shower as you would normally do, but be sure to use a mild cleansing lotion and a mild shampoo. You will be surprised by how the remaining protective film from the oil will keep your skin from drying out. Your skin will feel as soft as velvet throughout the entire day. Your hair will also look healthy and have a silky shine.

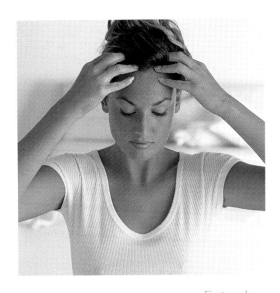

1 Oil yourself from head (entire head!) to toe. By the time you start with the massage, the oil will already be well absorbed.

2 Massage your head with your fingertips, as if you were shampooing your hair.
• "Shampoo" your entire scalp slowly and attentively, starting at the front hairline, moving over the sides and the top toward the back of your head, and then going all the way down to the neck.

3 The following is the ear massage, which lasts only ten seconds:
• Take both earlobes between the thumb and the index finger of both hands, and rub them delicately between your fingers.

4 Now you will gently massage your face:
- Place your fingertips at the center of your forehead, and while applying slight pressure pull the fingers left and right toward the temples. Conclude there with three circular motions. (Repeat this massage three times.)

Massage your face with long strokes and circular motions.

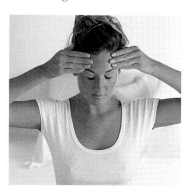

- Let your fingertips continue with the circular motions over your cheeks and down to your chin. From the chin, apply horizontal strokes the same way that you did on the forehead. (Repeat this massage three times.)
- Place both index fingers on the left and right sides of your nose, and stroke six times up and down.

5 Next comes the neck and the throat:
- Place your hands on your left and right shoulders, and rub them. Continue rubbing, while applying moderate pressure,

Rub the neck and the throat.

over the neck toward the hairline. Move up and down in this manner. (Repeat this massage six times.)
- At the throat, use both hands interchangeably to gently rub from the collarbone up to the chin. (Repeat this massage three times.)

6 Now massage the right arm, then the left:
- Massage the shoulder joint with small, circular motions on the skin. Stroke the upper arm with strong upward and downward motions. At the elbow, rub again with gentle circular motions; follow this by stroking the forearm, and conclude with a circular massage at the wrist.
- Carefully and gently stroke every finger, from the base of the fingers to the fingertips.
- Repeat this massage three times for each arm.

Massage the arms with strokes and circular motions.

7 Gently massage the chest with circular strokes. Women should massage around the breasts. (Repeat this massage three times.)

Gently stroke the chest with circular motions.

8 Lay your right hand flat on your stomach, while the left hand rests at the side of the body. With your right hand, make small, circular stroking motions over the skin in a clockwise direction, and then

gradually allow the circles to get larger, until the circular motion massages the entire stomach area.
● Let your right hand relax, and apply the same circular motions with the left hand.

9 A self-massage for the back is only possible on the lower back.

Rub the lower back and the buttocks forcefully.

● Stand up. Place your hands on the lower part of your back, and stroke it forcefully up and down.
● Massage your buttocks with the same motions.
● Repeat each of the above massages three times.

10 In order to massage your legs, you can sit down again now.

Massage the legs with circular motions and long strokes.

● Employ the same technique that you used in massaging your arms. But start at the bottom and work your way up.
● Repeat the massage three times per leg.

11 The feet are especially important because of their reflex points. Start by massaging the right foot, and then move over to the left foot. While massaging the feet, rest the calf on the opposite knee.
● Place one hand on the back of the foot and the other on the sole of the foot. Gently stroke

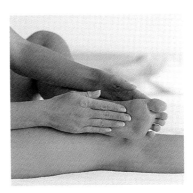

Stroking the feet

the foot, from the toes to the ankle and back again. (Repeat this massage three times.)
● Place both thumbs next to each other at the heel on the sole side of the foot. Run small spirals along this area with a degree of force. The spirals should progress toward your toes. Once you have reached your toes, release the pressure from your thumbs and let them glide back to the starting position. (Repeat this massage three times.)

Rubbing spirals on the sole of the foot

● Support your foot with one hand, and massage every toe separately, using small rubbing motions that proceed from the ankle joint to the tip of the toe. Carefully pull on each toe.
● Massage the skin between the toes by pressing the skin together and then pulling it.

Massaging the toes and the skin between the toes

For a Relaxed, Fresh Appearance

Our faces often look younger after a few massages, because wrinkles that were caused by tension have been smoothed away in a natural manner. A ten-minute facial massage can already be enough to get the blood circulation going and stimulate the lymphatic flow. Such a massage makes our complexions look fresh and prevents us from having puffy eyes.

Removes wrinkles that are caused by tension, and causes swelling to go down

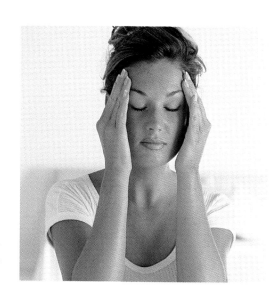

Gentle Facial Self-Massage

You can do the facial massage either in the morning as part of your grooming or in the evening if you still have plans and want to look fresh. You can also do it in between during your workday, which will then help you concentrate better.

➤ For "Massage Preparation," see page 31. Sit in a comfortable position, and spread a teaspoon of warm oil between your hands (see box on opposite page).

1 Lay your hands over your face for a few seconds, with your fingers on your forehead and the base of your hands on your chin.

Close your eyes, and breathe in and out deeply a few times.

2 Move your hands simultaneously to the left and the right, toward your ears. While making this motion, think of wiping away all the tension from your face, from your entire head, and from your spirit.
• Repeat this motion three times.

Cover your face with both hands, keep them there for a while, and then wipe away all tension.

3 Lay your hands on top of each other, horizontally, on the forehead. With both hands, gently stroke interchangeably in an upward motion over the forehead, from the ridge of the nose to the hairline. Close your eyes in order to truly enjoy this massage.
• Repeat the massage six times.

Stroking upward on the forehead

4 Place the fingertips of both hands between the eyebrows. Apply moderate pressure with fingers, and pull back in short, strong lines along the skin up toward your forehead. In this way, you can undo the little furrows in your forehead that are caused by creasing your eyebrows.

•Repeat this massage six times.

5 Stroke with the fingertips from the middle of the forehead toward the temples. At the temples, rub small circles in the skin, using as much pressure as feels comfortable for you.

•Slide your fingers back to the middle of the forehead, in order to pull them outward again.

•Repeat this massage a total of four times.

6 Press your eyebrows between the thumb and the index finger of both hands, from the middle toward the outside.

•Slide your fingers back, and lay your fingertips on the bridge of the nose, between the eyebrows. Applying moderate pressure, pull on the arc of the eyebrows by pushing them upward with half-circular motions. This stroke helps ease the tension in the area of your eyes and forehead.

•Repeat this massage a total of four times.

7 Place your fingertips to the left and the right sides of the nose. Apply moderate pressure, and stroke with your fingers to the side, over the cheeks, toward the ears.

•From the ears, glide your hands over to the corners of your mouth. From there, stroke again toward the outside, then back toward the tip of your chin, and from there, stroke over the lower jaw and back toward the neck.

•Repeat this massage three times.

8 Now cover your face with your hands, and stroke gently outward (breathing out) and then inward (breathing in).

For Additional Pleasure

•Sweet almond oil is recommended as the basic massage oil. If you add a drop of rose oil or neroli oil to 30 ml (2 tablespoons) of sweet almond oil, not only will it smell great but it will also have additional grooming and relaxing benefits.

•A facial sauna after a massage adds to the relaxing effect, and afterward the skin looks rosy and tight. Bring a quart (or liter) of water to a boil, let it cool down slightly, and add a teaspoon of rose water (which you can buy at your local health food store or drugstore). Keep your face above the steaming water for five minutes.

Massage for Cellulite

There is no wonder remedy.

There is no wonder cure for cellulite, even if the cosmetic industry is constantly promising one. The unattractive dents and thickening of the skin, which mostly occur in the thighs and on the buttocks, are caused by an accumulation of water and waste products in the fat cells of the connective tissue (see page 20). It is primarily women who have this problem, because the connective tissue in women is more capable of stretching.

Helpful Tips

There are several things you can do to prevent cellulite from forming and to reduce the appearance of already existing cellulite:
• Move around a lot on a regular basis. Aerobic exercise, jogging, walking, bicycling, and ballet are especially effective.
• Drink at least 2 quarts (or liters) of water a day. Green tea also has a purifying and preventive effect.
• Massage the problematic areas on a regular basis, preferably every morning.
• The following massage oils are recommended: aloe vera oil (this grooms the skin and also detoxifies), macadamia nut oil (this grooms the skin and gives a new firmness to dry, tired skin), jojoba oil (this grooms the skin, has no scent, and stays fresh for a long time), and "mature" sesame oil (see page 48).

Connective Tissue Massage for Problem Areas

Effective self-massage

The special gripping techniques of connective tissue massage create a strong stimulation along the skin and the connective tissue and thereby help accumulated water and fat to dissolve over time.

Due to the fact that cellulite mostly appears on the thighs and the buttocks, these areas are massaged with short, strong, directed strokes as well as with the so-called rolling grips, which are often very painful. Because of the pain associated with these motions, don't forget to breathe, as this will help you bear the pain.

Do not use this method if you have varicose veins.

➤ See "Massage Preparation" starting on page 31. You should stand while massaging the buttocks and sit while massaging the thighs.

1 First, spread some warm oil over the problem areas. Do not use an excessive amount of oil; you don't want your fingers to slide around too much.

Spread the oil

2 Place the index finger and the middle finger of both hands on the lower edge of your buttocks.
• Apply some pressure with your fingers, and pull them very slowly

Pull the buttocks with some force.

from the inside toward the outside. In other words, pull the fingers from the middle of your buttocks toward the hips. Then glide the fingers back again, while pulling in opposite directions, for a total of three times.
• Place your fingers a little higher up, and work all the way through the buttocks the same way. Each stroke in this massage should be applied three times.

Pull on the buttocks.

3 The following is a very effective pulling massage for the buttocks:
• You lift the skin with the fingertips of both hands, push it together slightly, and pull it upward. Then you let go and grab another area. You should apply this pulling technique to the entire problem area rapidly and forcefully.

4 For the following rolling massage, sit down on the floor (place a mat and a towel underneath your body!). The right leg will be treated first. Stand your right leg up, while the left one stays tucked underneath.
• Lift the skin with the thumb and the other fingers (at a right angle to the leg), and roll the tissue slowly against the fingers. In this manner, work your way slowly from the groin area toward the knee.

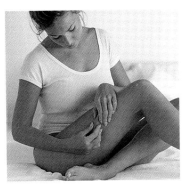

"Roll" the skin on the thigh . . .

. . . and then pull on it.

• When you come to the knee, lay the fingertips on the skin and pull them again in an upward motion toward the groin. Massage the entire area that has cellulite in this manner, first in a rolling motion and then in a pulling motion, all the while working your way from the hip to the knee.
• Depending on your threshold of pain, repeat this massage up to three times.
• Then move over to the left leg. Place the left leg up for the massage, and bend the right leg.

5 Complete the massage by calming down the area with a pleasant swinging motion. Lay your fingertips on the skin, and apply fast strokes in wavy motions (see page 29).

Complete the massage with a swinging motion.

Fitness Remedy for Muscles

Massage keeps the muscles elastic and strong, so that they will be ready for a high level of performance. This is why many professional athletes go to a massage therapist on a regular basis before and after training or during competitions. Massage helps to prevent muscles from cramping. It also helps in easing tension in cramped muscles and in providing a speedy recovery for injured muscles.

Please note those instances in which massage is not advised (page 68).

Whether you are a professional athlete or a weekend warrior, you can prevent possible injuries and muscular pain and tension by applying the simple grips that are presented here.

Some Other Tips

• Before engaging in any athletic activity, it's important to go through a ten-minute warm-up. By slowly stretching the individual muscles, you can make the muscles more elastic and also help prevent injuries.
• After your workout, take a ten-minute bath with a lavender bath supplement (which you can buy at your local health food store or drugstore) to prevent muscle spasms and help regenerate the muscles.

Self-Massage after Sports

The first step in the massage is especially effective after those athletic activities that turn around the axis of the body, such as tennis or golf.

➤ See "Massage Preparation" starting on page 31. You will need a tennis ball for this massage. To start, lie down comfortably on your back.

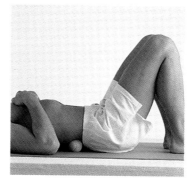

Place the tennis ball to the side of the spine, on the musculature in your lower back.

1 Bend your legs, placing your feet on the floor. Slightly lift your buttocks, and lay the tennis ball on the lower-left muscular area of your back, next to the spine (not directly under the spine!).

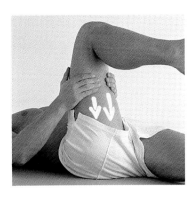

Massage the entire back with the assistance of a tennis ball.

- Slowly lower your back, and lay more and more body weight on the ball, as long as this remains comfortable. Hold this position for a while.
- Then lift the buttocks and push the tennis ball barely an inch (or a few centimeters) upward. Again, let your back down and stay in this position for a few seconds.
- In this manner, continue to massage your lower back, all the way up to the point directly below the shoulder blades.
- Then repeat the same massage on the right side of the spine.

The leg and arm massages can be used in conjunction with sports.

First massage the right thigh.

2 For the next step, start with the back of the right thigh:
- While lying down, bend the right knee, while the left leg remains stretched out. Grasp the right thigh with both hands directly at the knee.
- Apply pressure with your fingers, and pull both hands, at the same time, down toward the buttock.
- Allow your hands to gently glide back; then repeat these deep, effective strokes for a total of three times.

- Repeat the same procedure with the left thigh.

3 Next, massage the front of the thigh while sitting:
- Bend the left leg, while the right leg is stretched out. Lay your right hand flat over the knee, on the right thigh. Press with the left hand on the right hand, and make slow stroking motions this way, from the knee up toward the groin.
- Let both hands glide back

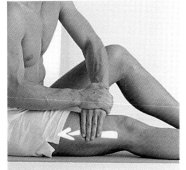

gently, and repeat this stroke three times.

4 Massage the inner side of the thigh the same way. Repeat this massage three times.
● Then massage the outer side of the leg (three times).
● Next, move over to the left leg.

5 Massaging the calf can be very painful when your muscles are cramped.
● While sitting, place one leg up, while the other lies bent to the side.
● Knead the calf musculature of the leg that is standing up—

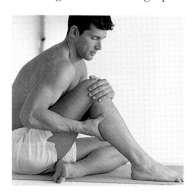

either gently or with force (it does not have to hurt!). Start at the heel, and work your way up to the hollow behind the knee.
● Let your hands glide back, and repeat the kneading motion three times, from the heel to the

hollow behind the knee.
● Next, change over to the other leg.

6 After the kneading, the calf musculature should be relaxed. You can relax the legs further by shaking the calves:
● While sitting, stand your legs up in a relaxed manner, on the heels. Hold each calf in one hand, and shake them back and forth for about a second.

7 Now we come to the arms. You can massage the arms either standing up or sitting down.
● Gently bend one arm, and lay the massaging hand beneath the shoulder, on the triceps.
● Work the triceps barely an inch (a centimeter) at a time, alternating between the application of pressure and release.

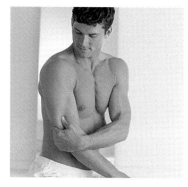

Massaging the forearm

• Next, place your hand below the elbow, on the musculature of the forearm, and massage the muscles using the same technique.

• Repeat all the grips at least three times, before changing over to the other arm.

8 The biceps are massaged the same way:

Massaging the biceps

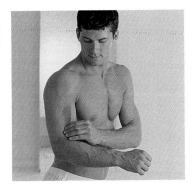

• Grasp the muscle above the elbow, with the thumb inside and the remaining fingers on the outside. Through pressure and release, slowly massage the arm all the way to the shoulder.

9 To complete the massage, stroke quickly downward, skipping the elbow, going over the muscles of the forearm; then stroke the arm quickly upward (again, skipping the elbow), all the way to the shoulder.

Stroking the forearm and the upper arm

• Repeat this massage on both arms at least ten times.

First Aid for Cramps in the Calves

If you tend to get cramps in your calves while or after participating in sports, or during the normal course of a day, you can release this tension quickly with a few simple hand grips:

1 Sit down, and stretch out the leg that hurts.

• With one hand, pull the leg as close as you can to your body, so that the calf is stretched out as much as possible.

Stretching and kneading the muscle of the calf

• Keep the leg in this position with that hand; at the same time, with the other hand, knead the calf as forcefully as possible, working your way from the bottom of the calf to the top of the calf.

2 When you feel that the muscle is beginning to release, stroke the entire leg with both hands. Stroke rapidly and rhythmically, from the foot, over the calf to the thigh, all the way up to the hip.

Stroking the entire leg

• The strokes that go up the leg should be administered with strong pressure, whereas the strokes that glide back down should be applied with gentle pressure.

Knead and stroke the leg until the cramp completely releases and the pain is relieved.

Duration

Gentle Massage for Babies

Most parents instinctively massage their babies—gentle caresses are a natural part of daily care. "It is as important to nourish a child with caresses and to nurture his skin and his back as it is to fill up his stomach." These words of the famous French obstetrician Frederic Leboyer clearly show that baby massage is not only effective for the skin but it is also a form of nurturing for babies and young children.

Healing Tender Loving Care

An extra portion of attention that is very effective.

Baby massage is an extra portion of attention that also has relaxing and healing effects:
• When children cry a lot and are irritated, the massage helps to relax their little organisms.
• Stomachaches or flatulence can be relieved effectively with your help.
• Many studies have shown that regular baby massages support the process of weight gain. Babies that are born prematurely need a lot of caress-ing not only to gain weight but also for the stimulation of various bodily functions, such as breathing and digestion; furthermore, caressing supplies the need for human contact, which is so crucial to the baby's survival.

Touching is a necessity of life.

Important Points to Remember While Massaging Your Child

• The room in which the massage takes place must be warm. The temperature should be at least 75 to 78 degrees F (or 24 to 26 degrees C). In the case of very small babies, it is recommended that you place an additional heater in the room to protect them from catching a cold.
• The duration of the baby massage should never be longer than ten minutes.
• Touch your baby with warm hands only. And make sure that you touch your baby gently, so that you don't scare it.
• The best time for the baby massage is between meals, because your baby should not have a full stomach during the massage, nor should it be hungry.
• If the child has a fever or an infection, you should not give it a massage.

The Baby Massage

You can integrate the baby massage into your daily care program without much inconvenience. You will readily see that your baby enjoys being massaged and is always happy when you lovingly pamper its body.

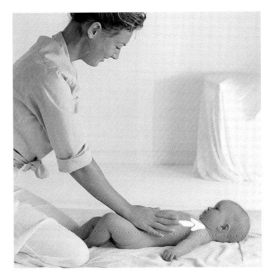

➤ Please note the recommendations on pages 31 and 32 as well as on the opposite page. Prepare some warm massage oil. The following are a selection of appropriate oils: sweet almond oil, aloe vera oil, and jojoba oil. You can also simply use baby oil.

The preparation

Lay your baby on the changing table, on a crawling blanket, or between your bent legs on a towel.

To start the massage, lay your baby on its back. This is important, because this way your baby can maintain eye contact with you.

1 Rub some massage oil into your hands, and lay your hands on your child's shoulders.

Stroking the upper body

- Gently apply even strokes from the shoulders outward, down the arms, all the way to the hands.
- Briefly hold the hands.
- Then lay your hands on the little stomach, and stroke

upward, over the ribcage, to the shoulders.
- Repeat this massage three times.

2 Enclose one of your baby's hands in one of your own hands in order to stabilize the arm. With the other hand, gently stroke from the forearm upward toward the upper arm and all the way to above the shoulder.
- Then gently stroke back down with that hand. (Repeat this massage three times.)
- Massage the other arm of your baby the same way.

3 Hold your baby's wrist with one hand. With the fingertips of the other hand, stroke over the back of your baby's

Gentle stroking has a calming effect, relaxes the muscles, and stimulates blood circulation.

Massaging the little arms

Massaging hands and fingers

hand to the fingertips. With every stroke over the back of the hand, gently knead another finger.

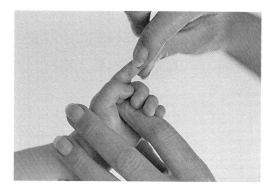

• Repeat this massage three times.
• Then switch to your child's other hand.

Stroking the little legs

4 Hold one of your baby's feet, and stroke it out with your other hand, over the calf, all the way to the hip.
• Next, gently glide your hand back to the foot. (Repeat this massage three times.)
• Repeat the same process with the opposite leg.

Massaging the feet and toes

5 With one hand, stabilize your child's foot. With the fingertips of your other hand, stroke over the back of the foot all the way to the toes, and with each stroke, knead another toe, just as you did with the hands.

➤ In order to massage the back of your baby, slowly turn the baby over onto its stomach. Babies can also have tense backs, so your baby will surely enjoy this back massage. Pay attention to massaging only the back muscle, not the spine!

Carefully lay your baby on its stomach.

6 Rub some massage oil into your hands, and lay your hands on the little buttocks.
• From there, stroke upward, over the back, to the shoulders. Gently grasp the shoulders, and let your hands rest there for a moment.
• Let your hands glide back to the buttocks, and repeat this stroke two more times.
• With the next upward motion, apply more massage strokes to the sides of the back by letting your hands glide over the outer sides of the body all the way up to the shoulders. At the shoulders, let your hands rest, and then let them glide down to the thighs. (Repeat this massage three times.)

Stroking the little back

7 Lay both your hands diagonally on your baby's back— one behind the other on the upper back—at the height of the shoulder blades.
• Start massaging by applying flowing, rhythmical strokes

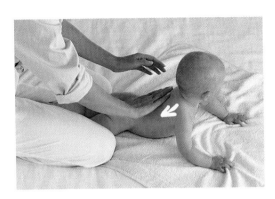

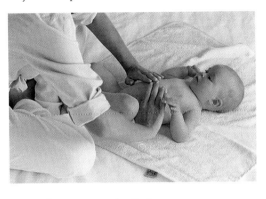

1 Spread some oil between your warm hands. Lay your hands on the right and left sides of your child's stomach, so that your fingertips rest over the belly button. Let your hands stay in this position for a while.

Calming the little stomach

Stroking the back with both hands inter-changeably down toward the buttocks. Always lift one hand after the other.

• If your child seems to enjoy this stroke, repeat it three times.

First Aid for Stomach-aches and Flatulence

Babies sometimes suffer from the acute abdominal pain of "three-month colic," and it is not unusual for babies and young children to have stomachaches and flatulence. Therefore, try to keep your baby from eating any food that creates gas (this goes for you, as well, in the event that you are breast-feeding).

Try to find out if your baby has an allergy.

Stomachaches and flatulence are occasionally related to an allergic reaction, so this would be worth investigating. The stomach massage with olive oil or Saint-John's-wort oil can be helpful in easing the pain.

• Start by pressing the little stomach muscles very gently and then letting them go. Be sure to make only very small and barely noticeable motions. Observe your child while doing this. If your child appears to like this gentle kneading, you can continue for about another minute. But if not, switch to the following grip:

Gently pressing and letting go

2 Stroke with the right hand in a clockwise direction around the belly button, while the left hand rests by the side. This calming motion has a pain-relieving effect, which makes it good for colic and stomachaches.

Stroking over the stomach in a clockwise direction

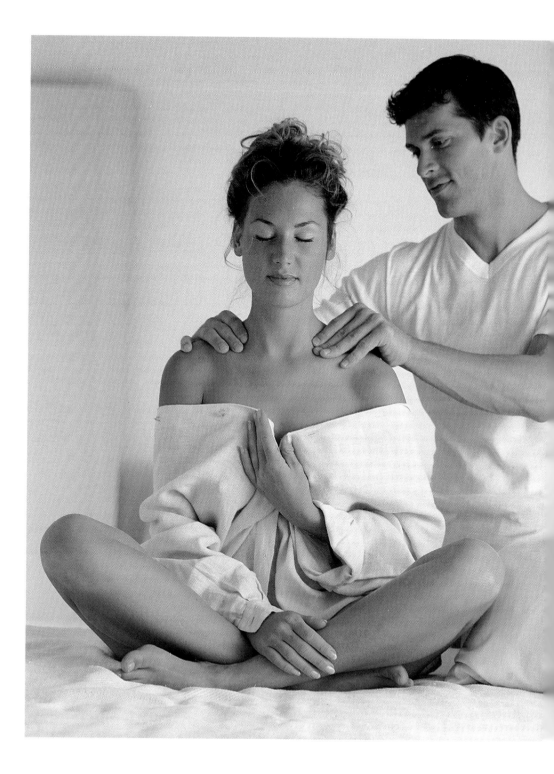

Helping and Healing with Massage

Whether you want to get rid of headaches or intestinal disorders, stabilize your circulation or do something to combat your sleeping problems, or ease the burdens that occur during pregnancy and childbirth—all this is possible with specific massages. Use the healing agencies of massage in your daily life—at home or at work. You will feel the effects: regular massages keep you healthy, prevent diseases, and heal many common complaints—and they do all this without any side effects!

The Alternative for Everyday Problems

There are days when you simply may not feel very well. You may have a headache, your circulation may seem a bit sluggish, or the constant pressure that you are under may be preventing you from getting a good night's sleep. The reasons for these annoying problems are not necessarily complicated or organic. It is possible that your physical and mental balance has been disturbed and this has manifested itself in physical symptoms.

When the inner balance is disturbed

Daily stress, responsibilities, the pressure of too many appointments, and sudden blows of fate can all cause a similar disturbance in our balance, as when we are sad, worried, mourning, or afraid, all of which are part of life, as are the beautiful, happy moments. It is especially in regard to these "negative states" that massage can be so beneficial. It can relieve many symptoms and help us achieve an inner balance.

Massage Instead of Medications

Most of us tend to turn to medications too quickly. This is seen in the constantly rising sales of over-the-counter drugs. In fact, digestion stimulants, sleeping pills, painkillers, and circulation stabilizers are among the best-selling products at many drugstores. However, the truth is that we could drastically reduce our consumption of medication through the application of massage.

Quickly grabbing tablets

Relieving Pain

The next time you are tempted to take a painkiller for a pressure headache, backache, neck pains, or menstrual cramps, first try to ease the pain through the regular application of massage. In addition to relieving pain, massage leads to an overall sense of well-being.

It is worth your while to give it a chance!

Sleeping Better

All sleeping aids have a negative effect on our physical and mental states, regardless of their herbal or chemical origin. In extreme cases, we can even become addicted to these drugs. For these reasons, look for the underlying cause of your sleeping problem before you turn to medication. Often it is physical and emotional tension that robs us of a good night's sleep. Relaxing massages support our ability to fall asleep and to sleep through the night, and if they are applied on a regular basis they can give us the gift of recovery through a good, sound sleep (see page 38).

Relaxation helps sleep.

Stabilizing Circulation

Improved blood circulation

Dizziness while getting up, tiredness, difficulties concentrating, or having chronically cold hands and cold feet—all are signs that our circulation is out of balance. Massage has the ability to stimulate blood circulation, so that it becomes unnecessary to take medications (see page 14).

Stimulating the Intestines

Stomach and intestinal problems are very common. Most people seek help through medications that stimulate digestion. But just as is the case with sleeping aids, these medications are effective only when they are taken on a regular basis. The intestines get used to the medications, however, and gradually decrease their level of activity.

Remove the causes as well.

A low level of intestinal activity and a variety of discomforts, including heartburn and feeling bloated, can often be due to eating the wrong foods and not getting enough exercise.

Targeted massages (see page 80) can reactivate the intestines. In addition, think about changing your diet and be sure to get regular exercise.

Help with Pregnancy and Birth

Frequent massages during pregnancy help alleviate back pain, insomnia, and recurring muscle spasms. As long as your pregnancy is not in danger, and your gynecologist has not cautioned you against receiving massages, most of the massages in this book can be applied over the course of your pregnancy. *The only massage that you should not receive during pregnancy is the foot reflexology massage, because it is so intense.*

Pay attention to this!

During the actual childbirth, it is also helpful to receive loving caresses, especially in the lower-back area. They ease the process of giving birth as well as alleviate the feelings of fear and fatigue often associated with it.

After the birth, massages stimulate the physical and mental recovery of the mother (anti-stress massages, page 38) and speed up the regeneration pro-cess (stomach massage, page 80).

The Limits of Self-Treatment

Massage is not always the right solution. Even though massage is very effective in a broad spectrum of ways, it is sometimes limited in its ability to solve certain problems. This is especially true in the case of chronic, recurring, or acute problems. You need be aware that there are certain diseases or conditions that should not be treated with massage and that there are others that should only be treated by a professional massage therapist. It's also important to know that massage therapy is allowed for certain complaints although the possibilities of its use in these cases must first be discussed with the patient's doctor.

Contraindications

Massage therapy should not be applied in the following cases:
- Acute infections, such as infections of the kidneys, veins, bones, and joints
- Acute injuries to the tendons, ligaments, and muscles
- A slipped disc
- Bone diseases, such as osteoporosis or joint tuberculosis
- Diseases of the vascular system, such as thrombosis
- Diseases involving a widening of the blood vessels (aneurysm), severe varicose veins
- Fever
- Cancer
- Heart diseases
- Freezing and burning

You should seek the *advice of a doctor* in the following cases:
- Skin diseases (also infections under the skin), varicose veins
- Diabetes mellitus
- Pregnancy (especially in the case of a risky pregnancy)

These cases should only be treated by a *professional massage therapist*:
- Sciatica
- Throat, breast, and lumbar vertebra syndromes
- Rheumatism
- Neurological diseases, such as paralysis
- Consequences of injuries and operations on the moving apparatus
- Internal disorders, such as heart problems and high blood pressure
- Children whose physical development is impeded in some manner

Relaxation for the Head and Back

Headaches

Massaging the face and the head gives us a general feeling of relaxation. The face and head massage can be especially helpful for those people who tend to solve everyday problems by "only using their heads." This solely intellectual attitude leads to all kinds of tension in the head area.

Our skulls are covered with a very thin layer of muscle that reacts to emotional tension by developing cramps. But there are also other reasons for headaches, such as too little physical movement or an oxygen deficiency, consuming too much alcohol or nicotine, and sudden changes in the weather as well as extreme weather conditions.

The face and head massage can help in alleviating:
- Headaches caused by tension
- Migraines
- Fatigue and general pressure
- Lymphatic blockages in the face
- Colds and sinus problems (without fever)

Tension, stress, and other causes

Massage helps in all of these cases.

A Tip for Relieving Headaches

Peppermint oil can be as effective in alleviating headaches as any painkiller. This has even been proven scientifically.

Mix 1 teaspoon of sunflower oil with 1 drop of peppermint oil, and rub the mixture on the forehead, temples, and neck.

The Face and Head Massage

See "Massage Preparation" starting on page 31. If you are performing a partner massage, your partner should be lying down comfortably and be covered with a blanket in order to stay warm. You should be kneeling down or sitting behind your partner's head.

You can also apply this massage to yourself. If this is the case, sit at a desk or a table, with your feet flat on the floor and your elbows supported on the desk or the table.

Use only a little warmed-up oil (see page 38), because the surface for the application of this massage is very small.

As a partner massage or a self-massage

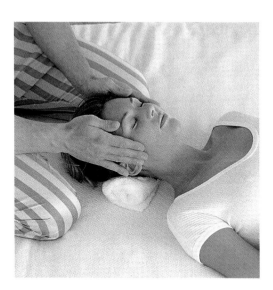

2 Lay the fingertips of both hands flat on the middle of the forehead.
- Rub ten to fifteen circles on the skin, while applying gentle pressure.
- Next, start making spiral motions toward the temples, until you arrive at the temples themselves.

Massage the forehead with circular motions.

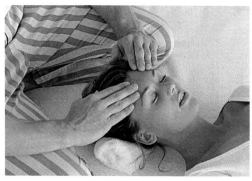

Gently establish contact by stroking the face.

1 Establish contact with flowing, gentle strokes, spreading the oil evenly over the entire face:
- Lay your hands protectively over the throat and the chin. Stroke with both hands, while applying slight pressure, toward the ears and beyond, and then over the cheeks to the temples. While doing this, feel the contours of the face and simply allow your hands to glide over the surface.
- From the temples, stroke with your fingers toward the middle of the forehead. Let your fingers meet there and rest for a while, and then glide your fingers back over the temples to the chin.
- Repeat the entire process three times.

- Once you arrive at the temples, rub another ten circles there.
- After a few seconds, move your fingers in small spiral motions over the cheeks toward the nose, and from there move them at an angle down toward the jaw.
- The fingers meet at the chin, where they rub ten more circles.
- Next, hold the face with both hands, and let your hands glide up to the center of the forehead.
- From this point, repeat the rubbings two more times.

Apply circular motions, passing over the temples, the cheeks, and the chin.

3 Gently press both eyebrows between the thumb and the index finger of both hands, and then let them go. Knead the curve of the eyebrows less than half an inch (a centimeter) at a time, starting at the nose and

Knead the eyebrows . . .

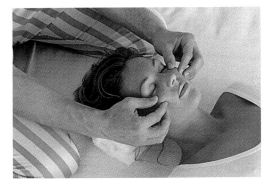

. . . and the cheeks.

lobes, and continue upward all the way to the upper edges. Do this slowly, moving up a little bit at a time.
Repeat this motion three times.

Kneading the ears

6 Lay your fingertips on the forehead, and stroke up toward the hairline.
• Next, grasp the hair with the fingers, and pull gently on the hair and let go. Then grasp another spot, repeating the same process over and over with all the hair on the scalp.

Pull gently on the hair of the scalp.

moving out to the temples.
• Afterward, knead the cheek muscles with your fingertips. Start at the nose, and knead all the way to the ears, and from there, continue in an angle down toward the jaw.
• Allow your fingertips to glide up to the eyebrows; then repeat the kneading motion two more times.

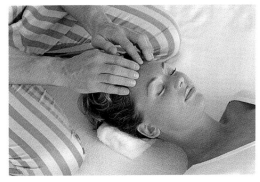

Envelop the face.

4 Cover the face with both hands, and wait a few seconds before beginning the ear massage.

5 Knead the ears between the index finger and the thumb of both hands. Start at the ear-

7 Lay your fingertips on the front part of the hairline, and then rub the skin of the entire scalp with strong, circular motions, as if you were shampooing.

Massaging the skin of the scalp with circular motions

8 Finally, lay your hands over the face again for about a minute. While doing this, breathing should be calm and even.

Tension in the Neck and Shoulders

The neck and shoulders area frequently tends to get tense. This is because many muscles that are constantly working and often pressured improperly converge here.

Frequent problems with various causes People who are overweight and work sitting down are especially prone to having bad posture, which can lead in the worst case to the so-called neck-spine syndrome. The first signs of this syndrome are headaches, painful tension in the neck and shoulders, and a tingling feeling and numbness in the hands.

A tense neck can also be caused by a chill due to air conditioning or by uncomfortable sleeping positions. However, sometimes tension can be the result of the fears that settle down in our necks or the feeling of having too much responsibility "on our shoulders." The regular application of the neck and shoulders massage can help ease the pain and return the muscles to a relaxed and smooth state.

The neck and shoulders massage is helpful for:
- Headaches caused by tense neck muscles
- Painful cramps of the neck and shoulder muscles
- A stiff neck accompanied by pain and limited mobility of the head
- Fear and the feeling of being overtaxed

Massage helps in all these cases.

The Neck and Shoulders Massage

➤ See "Massage Preparation" starting on page 31. Your partner can sit on a chair in a riding position, straddling the seat. Place a pillow on the back of the chair, so that your partner can rest his or her forehead on it (see page 45). However, the massage is more relaxing if applied while your partner is lying down (see page 34). At the beginning, you should be either standing, sitting, or kneeling next to your partner. During the final stage of the massage, you should be behind your partner's head.

The partner massage— for the self-massage, see page 42.

A Tip for a Stiff Neck

If you have a stiff neck, try this: Under warm running water in the shower, slowly and gently turn your head to the right and to the left, going a little further with every turn. After getting out of the shower, soak a towel in hot water, wring it out, lay it around your neck, and then take a dry towel and drape it around the wet towel. Now lie down and relax for ten minutes.

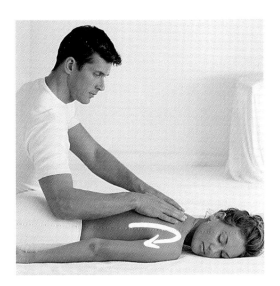

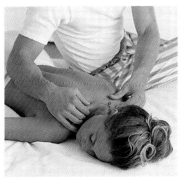

2 The following kneading massage can be very painful. Therefore, pay close attention to how your partner reacts. It shouldn't be too painful!
• Start by kneading the muscles on both shoulders at the same time for about a minute.

Kneading both shoulders simultaneously

• Relax the area with a wave-like swinging motion (see page 29).

Establishing contact through gentle strokes

1 Make contact through gentle strokes, while also spreading the massage oil:
• Cautiously, lay your hands to the left and to the right of the spine, at the height of the shoulder blades. By slightly leaning forward, you can add some pressure to your touch; then stroke upward, reaching the neck and then the back of the head.
• Next, glide your hands back down, on both sides of the neck, to the shoulders, and then further down the body, all the way to the upper arms. From there, swiftly stroke your hands back to the beginning position, between the shoulder blades.
• Repeat this flowing motion four times.

3 Continue by kneading only the right side with both hands. Slowly work your way from the shoulder to the hairline, less than a half inch at a time.
• From there, apply strong strokes with the tips of the fingers back toward the shoulder.
• Repeat the kneading massage two more times, and then massage the left side in the same manner.

Kneading and stroking one shoulder at a time

4 Lay both thumbs to the left and to the right of the spine, between the shoulder blades.

Rub in small circular motions on the skin, while applying moderate pressure. Slowly rub your way up to the hairline by interchanging between circular and spiral motions.

Make circles and spirals with the thumbs, beginning at the shoulder blades and going all the way up the neck, ...

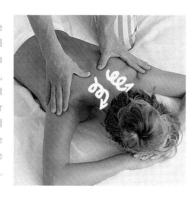

- When you get to the hairline, lay the tips of your thumbs flat on the hairline, apply some pressure, and hold them there for a few seconds. Release the pressure, and then move the thumbs away from each other, while applying some more pressure.

... and then massage the hairline.

- With this kind of massage—alternating between the application of pressure and release—slowly massage the entire hairline all the way up to the ears.
- Afterward, let your thumbs glide back to their original position, between the shoulder blades. Repeat this process three times.

5 Repeat Step 1 (gentle stroking) four times.

First Aid for Tension in the Neck

Even though the following massage is not administered with the hands, the "head rocking" massage is considered to be one of the most pleasurable kinds of massage.

By slowly turning the neck, the muscles there are stretched out in the best way possible. Cramps and tensions can be released in this manner, and the mobility of the neck increases while the pain disappears.

This partner massage is especially pleasant.

➤ You can do this massage before or after the neck and shoulders massage. Your partner lies comfortably on his or her back on a mat and is covered with a blanket. You need to have a towel, which you then spread beneath your partner's head. You should choose a comfortable position for yourself, either standing or kneeling down above your partner's head.

Before or after the neck and shoulders massage

1 Bend forward, and hold one end of the towel with each hand.
- Carefully lift the towel slightly, so that your partner's head is not resting on the mat but on the towel. Pay attention to be sure that the head is secure and resting comfortably on the towel.

Lifting the head with a towel

• Ask your partner to completely relax, breathe calmly, and let go of thoughts.

2 Slowly pull on the right side of the towel, so that your partner's head gradually turns left—as far as it can. Check to be sure that your partner is still comfortable. It is of utmost importance for your partner to

Turning the head by carefully pulling on the towel

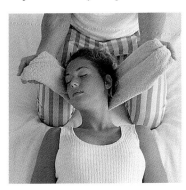

surrender to this movement; your partner shouldn't be turning his or her head—the turning should occur on its own. You should be very aware of this aspect of the massage and stop pulling right away if you feel that your partner is making the movements.

• Next, slowly bring the head back to the first position (the middle) by carefully pulling on the left side of the towel.

• Wait for a few seconds; then pull the towel further, so that the head can turn to the right side.

• Repeat this process three times.

Back Pain

Every third person in Germany suffers from back pain—a disturbing fact. It has been proven that people who have chronic back pain made certain mistakes over the course of many years. Perhaps they slept on mattresses that were too soft, wore the wrong shoes, sat for hours on chairs with poor back support, both at work and at home, exercised too little or too much (as in the case of professional athletes), ate the wrong foods, or were under constant stress.

Reasons for back pain

Mental and emotional states can also affect posture and cause back pain. For example, when we are sad or depressed, our posture will be affected, even though we might not be aware of this. Over time, bent posture can develop into constant muscular tension throughout the entire back. Persisting in keeping our "inner posture" upright against all odds can also cause back pain.

Often it is a manifestation of emotional problems.

When the back is overtaxed, for whatever reason, the back muscles harden with every stiff effort, and over time this can produce pain. In addition to a general change in lifestyle, reeducating the back, and exercising daily, regular back massages can help ease the pain in this area. They will relax the back muscles, while also helping the entire body and the soul to calm down.

Relieves the pain

The back massage is helpful in counteracting:
• Problems caused by spinal distortion (scoliosis)
• Minor problems with the sciatic nerve
• Back problems during pregnancy (see page 67)
• Back pain before or during menstruation
• Stress-related tension in the musculature of the back
• General states of fatigue and nervousness

Massage is helpful in these cases.

Tips for Maintaining a Healthy Back

Take a look at your lifestyle:
• If you are under constant stress, there are techniques for relaxation that can be helpful, such as visualizations and meditation.
• Make sure that you wear comfortable shoes. Narrow shoes or high heels can cause you to have tense posture and can burden the back.
• Activities that are good for the back include swimming on the back, gymnastics that involve the spine, yoga, and walking. Try doing at least one on a regular basis.

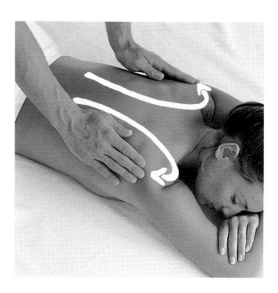

The Back Massage

➤ See "Massage Preparation" starting on page 31. You can find formulas for relaxing and pleasant massage oils on page 38.

It is important for your partner to be lying down comfortably. Small pillows and neck rolls are helpful (see page 34). Your partner should be naked and covered with a warm blanket. You should be kneeling down or standing next to your partner.

If your massage partner is pregnant, the back massage must be administered while she is in a seated position (see page 45) or lying on her side (see page 35).

This partner massage also begins with gentle strokes.

1 First, rub warmed massage oil between your hands.

Then place both hands on the lower back.

Stroking the back

- Apply some pressure to the hands by bending forward slightly. In a flowing motion, gently stroke the muscles along the left and the right sides of the spine upward toward the neck.
- From there, stroke over the shoulders to the sides of the back, and then let your hands glide down toward the buttocks. Next, lead them in a semicircle back inward, toward the spine.
- You are back in the starting position. From here, you can begin stroking upward again.
- Repeat this massage six times.

To work deeper, press the knuckles upward . . .

2 For a deeper massage, use the knuckles.
- Bend your fingers into half-open fists. Lay the backs of the fingers on the lower back,

to the left and to the right of the spine. Push both hands with pressure toward the neck.
- At the base of the neck, open your hands without losing contact with the skin, so that the palms of your hands are now placed on the skin.
- Stroke the outer sides of the back, over the shoulders and the shoulder joints, until you return once more to the lower back (the first position).
- Repeat this massage three times.

. . . and then stroke back with the palms.

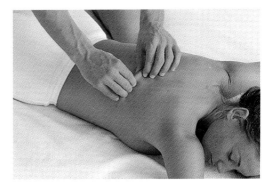

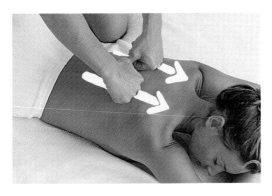

3 Knead only the muscles that are opposite you. In other words, if you are standing on the left side of your partner, you should first work the muscles on the right side of your partner's back. Then do the massage the other way around.
- To administer this massage, take both hands and press a fold of skin on the lower back,

Knead the muscles on both sides of the spine.

between the spine and the hip, and knead it through with care.
- Knead all the way up to the base of the neck; then let both hands glide back to the base of the lower back.
- Go through these kneading motions again, before you move to work on the other side.

4 By means of rubbing motions, you can detect and release small muscular tensions:
- Place both hands again on the lower back, and with slightly bent thumbs rub the muscles along both sides of the spine using small circular motions.

Rub in small circular motions with the thumbs along the sides of the spine.

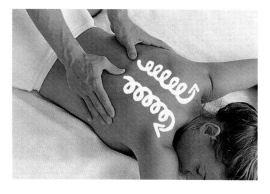

- Work your way up very slowly by creating a spiral and then rubbing in circular motions on the same spot for a few seconds.
- When you reach the base of the neck, let your hands glide back to the starting position on the lower back. Then repeat

these rubbing motions two more times.

5 If the back muscles are very tense, it would be a good idea to work both sides of the back again, but this time one after the other. Start again on the lower back:

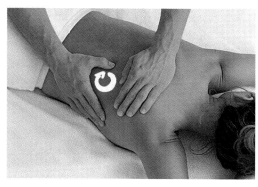

- Always place one hand in front of the treated area, while you rub small spiral motions in a clockwise direction on the skin with the other hand.
- Work your way up to the hairline in this manner very slowly. Once you reach the hairline, let your hands glide back.
- Repeat this massage two more times, before devoting yourself to the other side of the back.

Rub each side separately with the thumbs.

6 Complete the massage by repeating the gentle and deep strokes described in Step 1 and Step 2. Repeat each of the motions three times.

Complete the massage with strokes.

First Aid for the Back— Foot Reflexology You Can Do Yourself

The reflex zones of the back When no partner is around to relieve you of your back pain, a massage of the relevant foot reflex zones can be helpful (without massage oil!). As seen in the illustration, the reflex points on the back are located along the arch of the foot.

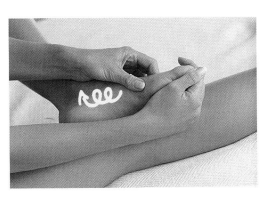

Rubbing the arch of the foot with circular motions

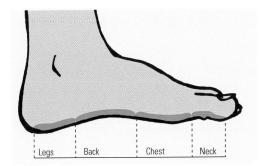

| Legs | Back | Chest | Neck |

➤ Sit comfortably, laying one foot across the thigh of the other leg.

• Stabilize the foot with one hand, while you lay the thumb of the other hand over the big toe below the first knuckle.

• Rub small spirals along the inner edge of the arch of the foot with your thumbs, while applying moderate pressure. Run these spirals toward the heel of the foot. Work very slowly. The places where you experience pain reflect the painful areas in your back. Devote special attention to these areas by continuously massaging spirals on them for ten seconds each.

• Once you reach the heel, stroke with the thumbs back toward the starting position.

• Repeat these rubbing motions two more times, before switching over to the other foot.

Tips for Enhancing the Massage

This will heighten the effectiveness of the massage: Take a warm foot bath (96 to 100 degrees F, or 36 to 38 degrees C). During the bath, do some assorted foot exercises: for example, spread your toes and widen and stretch your feet. Afterward, dry your feet and rub them with a healing and relaxing oil made from 3 drops of neroli oil in 2 table-spoons of almond oil.

Treating the Stomach and Intestines

Caressing the Stomach and the Soul

The entire area of the stomach is a highly sensitive part of the body that can be influenced easily by massage. The stomach massage has a harmonizing and relaxing effect and improves our overall sense of well-being. In cases of a low level of intestinal activity, the stomach massage can be so effective in regulating digestion that it may seem like magic. Menstrual cramps can be relieved with this type of massage.

Improves our overall well-being

Stomach Massage through Breathing

Consciously breathing into your stomach not only affects your general well-being, but all the stomach and digestive organs get massaged and stimulated as well. Breathe in through your nose, and pull the air down to the lower abdomen, so that the stomach expands. Then let the air flow slowly out of your mouth. Pause briefly, and then breathe in again in a relaxed manner. Repeat this process five times.

Use this technique several times a day, either lying down or standing up.

Problems in the stomach and intestinal area may have to do with an improper diet, eating too quickly, lack of physical movement, stress, or conflicts that are hard to "digest." Therefore, it is important to discover the causes and, if possible, to eliminate them as well.

Discovering the causes of the problem

The stomach massage is helpful in alleviating:
- Fear, inner unrest
- Nervous stomach
- Lack of appetite
- Digestion problems, such as constipation, feeling bloated, flatulence, stomach pressure, and an upset stomach
- Menstrual cramps

Massage is helpful in these cases.

The Stomach Massage

➤ See "Massage Preparation" starting on page 31. For formulas for relaxing massage oils, see page 38.

In order to perform a partner massage on the stomach area, your partner needs to lie down comfortably on his or her back (see page 34), and you should be standing up or kneeling down at your partner's side. For a self-massage, you should be lying

Appropriate as both a partner massage and a self-massage

down comfortably on your back. *Important:* Whoever will be receiving the stomach massage should not eat anything beforehand. It's also important not to drink very much. Massaging a full stomach can cause very unpleasant feelings and even lead to nausea.

1 Spread the warmed-up massage oil between your warm hands, and carefully place your hands on the lower abdomen.
• Allow the hands to rest there for a few seconds, in order to establish contact in a quiet and relaxed way.
• Afterward, apply some pressure and then stroke upward, over the stomach and the breastbone, toward the shoulders.

• From there, your hands glide back to the starting position.
• Repeat this massage three times.

2 Passively lay one hand on the lower ribs, to support the other hand.
• With the other hand, start

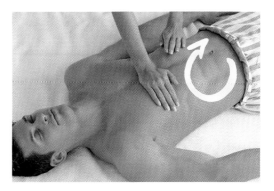

stroking in large circles in a clockwise direction, while applying gentle pressure. Begin the circles below the belly button.
• Repeat this motion ten times.

3 Place your hands on the right and left sides of the stomach, and create large circles with both hands in a clockwise direction:
• When the right hand pulls the circle downward, the left is stroking upward. As the circular motion continues, your hands cross each other. When this happens, lift the left hand

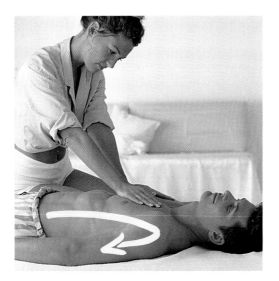

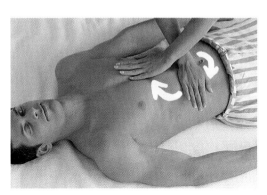

with strong wringing and drumming motions.

• Next, knead the abdominal wall with a gentler touch. Knead from the center of the body outward toward the right side of the waist, and then stroke gently with the finger-

Stroking with both hands crossed over the right hand, laying it back down on the stomach immediately.

• While lifting your hand and crossing it over, try to achieve a flowing rhythm with this motion, so that your partner— and you as well—will have the feeling that you are creating circular motions that are connected to each other.

• Repeat this process six times.

4 In order to stimulate blood circulation in the stomach muscles and relax them too, we use the technique of kneading on the entire stomach area.

You begin by treating the right side. In partner massage, you work the right side by being at your partner's left side (then you switch over to the other side).

• The "meaty" area at the sides *Massaging* of the waist are treated with *the waist by* both hands at the same time *"drumming"* by moving up toward the ribs

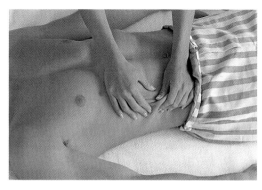

tips back toward the middle.

• Lay your fingers next to the area that was massaged already, and knead this area toward the waist. Work in this way over several rows across the stomach.

• Repeat the entire kneading process once more, and then switch over to the left side of the body.

Kneading the abdominal wall from the middle out to the side

5 Complete the stomach massage by repeating the strokes described in Step 1 and Step 3 three more times.

Completing the massage with more strokes

Relief for the Arms and Legs

The arms and the hands, as well as the legs and the feet, work hard on a daily basis. Our legs and feet must carry the entire weight of our bodies, while we master our daily tasks with numerous hand grips and arm movements.

During work and while participating in sports, great demands are placed on these parts of the body. Professions that require one to stand for many hours on end, as well as sports played by professional athletes, can bring about chronic problems in the musculature of the arms and the legs.

Wearing the wrong shoes plays just as large a role in the occurrence of cramps in the legs and the feet. In addition, a lack of movement, caused by sitting for extended periods of time, can lead to insufficient circulation of the blood in the muscles as well as to limp and untrained muscles. This in turn can lead to muscular cramps and stiff muscles.

Massaging the limbs is not only relaxing but can also help relieve many problems that are caused by overworking the muscles or not working them enough.

Massaging the limbs is helpful in easing:
• Tension in the musculature of the arms and the legs
• Muscular cramps
• Circulation problems (cold hands and cold feet)
• Swollen legs or swollen arms caused by extended periods of standing or sitting.

Easing Tension in the Arms and Hands

Often we are not aware of the tension that has developed in our hands and arms. A massage of these areas is a very relaxing and pleasant experience, easing tension that was created in a passive manner. Moreover, an inner ability to let go is heavily dependent on the relaxation of the parts of the body that are responsible for gripping and holding on.

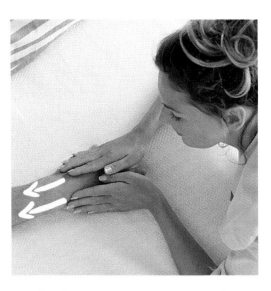

the elbow and then further, over the upper arm, all the way to the shoulder.
• Next, let your hands gently glide back to the original position.
• Repeat this massage four times.

2 Reinforce the pressure in your hands for the deep-tissue strokes:
• Hold the wrist from the outside with one hand and from the inside with the other.
• From the wrist, stroke upward in a forceful manner to the elbow. Once you reach the elbow, reduce the pressure for a

Start by stroking the hands and the arms.

Partner Massage for the Arms . . .

➤ See "Massage Preparation" starting on page 31. This massage will loosen up the arms and the shoulders. Your partner can lie on his or her back or sit on a comfortable chair with side arms. You should be kneeling down or sitting in front of the arm that you are going to treat.

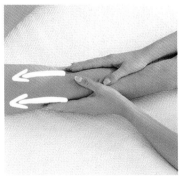

Applying deep-tissue strokes to the arm

Begin with gentle stroking.

1 Start with a gentle stroking massage on the right arm:
• Spread enough massage oil between your hands (up to a spoonful when the arms are very dry), and lay your hands on your partner's right arm.
• Stroke your partner's arm up to

second, and then continue forcefully stroking the upper arm.
• When you arrive at the shoulder joint, let your hands gently slide backward.
• Repeat this motion three times.

3 The following step is referred to as "kneading." Start at the shoulder joint. A

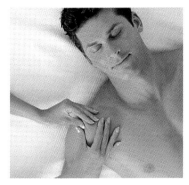

very important muscle covers this area: the deltoid muscle.
• Use the tips of all your fingers to knead the shoulder up to the base of the neck.
• From there, the fingertips glide back to the shoulder joint.
• Repeat this kneading motion two more times.

4 In order to knead the biceps in the front part of the upper arm, begin right above the elbow and knead upward to the shoulder joint. This time, you should press and knead only

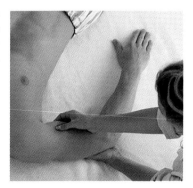

with the right hand, while the left hand supports the arm at the elbow joint.
• Gently stroke with the right hand back to the elbow, and then knead the triceps, which are located on the back of the upper arm. This time, it is the left hand that is working, while the right hand supports the arm at the elbow.
• Repeat the alternating kneading motion a total of three times.

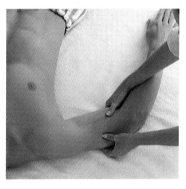

5 Now knead the lower area of the right arm with the same kind of alternating hand grips:
• While your left hand is supporting the forearm at the wrist, knead upward with the right hand along the inner side of the arm to the elbow.
• With a gentle stroke, allow the working hand to glide back to the wrist.
• At the wrist, change hands, so that you are now supporting with the right hand and knead-

Kneading the outer side of the forearm

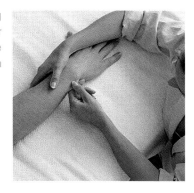

ing the outer side of the arm with the left hand.
• Repeat this massage three times

. . . and the Hands

Once again, start on the right side.

6 Hold the open hand of your partner with both of your hands. You partner's hand should be facing up.
• Lay both thumbs parallel to each other on the palm above the finger joints, and stroke with both thumbs at the same time toward the wrist.

Stroking the palm

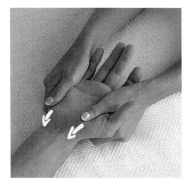

• Now the thumbs glide back, and then stroke up and down three more times.
• Next, rub small spirals on the skin, using both of your thumbs. Start again at the finger joints, and move up to the wrist.
• From there, gently stroke back

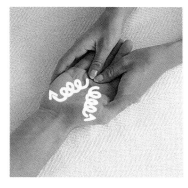

Rubbing in spiral motions

again, and repeat the rubbing motion three more times.

7 Carefully turn your partner's arm, so that his or her palm is lying in your hands.
• Now you will be massaging the muscles between the fingers by using both of your thumbs at the same time. You start the massage at the "webs" of the little fingers and the thumbs, and proceed by stroking your way up to the wrist.
• This step is followed by a gentle stroking motion in the reverse direction, placing your thumbs on the area between the ring finger and the index

Stroking the back of the hand

Stroking
between the
bones of the
fingers

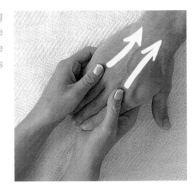

finger. From here, stroke upward again toward the wrist.
• Repeat the stroking of all the
areas in between the fingers for
a total of four times.

Massaging
every finger
individually

8 Support your partner's hand
with your left hand.
• Hold the thumb at the base
of the nail between your right
thumb and your index finger,
and roll it back and forth
between them.
• After a little while, take hold
of a slightly higher spot on the
thumb, and roll it back and
forth again between your thumb
and index finger. Continue to
slowly work your way up in this
manner until you reach the joint
of the thumb.
• Then massage the index finger, the middle finger, the ring
finger, and the little finger in the
same manner.
• It is recommended to massage each finger twice.

9 Complete the massage with
an upward stroke, which
has the effect of relieving tension and stimulating blood circulation.
• With one hand, hold your
partner's hand at the wrist,
and, with other hand, hold
your partner's forearm at
around the same height.
• Apply strong, flowing strokes
to the inside of the arm all the
way up to the shoulder joint.
While doing this, push the
skin ahead of you and apply

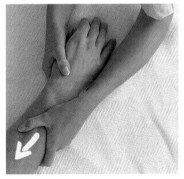

Strongly
stroking the
arm

pressure to the blood vessels.
• When you arrive at the
shoulder joint, allow your
hand to gently slide back.
• Apply this stroke two more
times.

10 After this, devote yourself to your partner's left
arm and left hand, repeating
Steps 1 through 9.

And now the
left arm and
the left hand

Working the Legs and Feet

Important: If your partner suffers from varicose veins, it is inadvisable for him or her to receive the leg massage. In the case of less severe problems, seek the advice of a doctor before you begin.

Not to be applied in cases of varicose veins

Partner Massage for the Legs . . .

➤ See "Massage Preparation" starting on page 31. The massage begins with your partner lying down on his or her stomach; later, your partner will have to turn over on his or her back. You should always be standing or kneeling down next

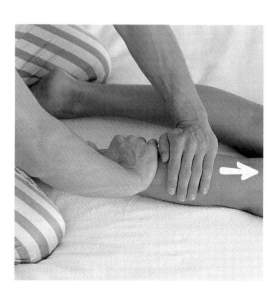

to the leg that is being massaged. When you administer the foot massage, you should be directly in front of the foot that you are treating.

Start the massage by gently stroking up the back of the leg.

For Beautiful Legs and Feet

• Run around barefoot often. Wear comfortable shoes, and change the pair of shoes that you are wearing on a daily basis.
• Perform athletic activities like swimming, cycling, and walking on a regular basis.
• Give up using the elevator or the escalator, and walk up the stairs instead.
• Take alternating foot baths (concluding with cold water) on a daily basis, in order to ensure good blood circulation.
• Eat a diet of whole foods that contain very little salt, and be sure to drink a lot of liquids (water and herbal tea).

1 The first step is to massage the back of the right leg:
• Spread massage oil between your hands (if the legs are very resistant, you will need a maximum amount of 2 spoonfuls), and place your hands over the ankle, with the fingertips toward the middle, crossed over each other.
• Hold the leg, and stroke it with both hands, with some applied pressure, up to the hollow of the knee, and then all the way up the thigh to the edge of the buttock.
• Once you are at the edge of the buttock, pull your hands away

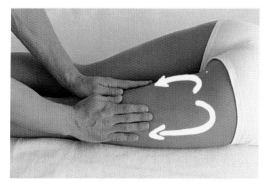

to the starting position. (Repeat this massage three times.)
- Then hold the leg at the hollow of the knee, and while the left hand is now passive, knead the muscles of the outer side of the leg up toward the buttock with the right hand.
- With a gentle downward stroke, glide back to the starting position. (Repeat this massage three times.)

Kneading the outer side

Stroking with the hands down the sides of the legs from each other and allow them to gently glide along the outside and the inside of the leg back down to the ankle.
- Repeat this massage six times.

3 Now prepare the calf for the massage by applying a series of deep-tissue strokes:
- Hold the leg with one hand at the ankle. Close the other

2 The following is the massage for the thighs:
- Hold the leg at the hollow of the knee with both hands. **Kneading the inner side of the leg** While the right hand remains still, slowly knead the inner side of the leg with the left hand up toward the buttock.

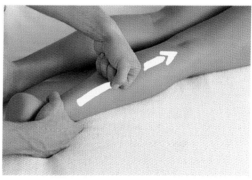

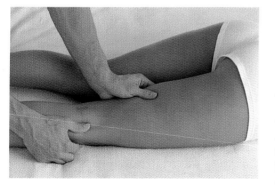

- From there, let your hand glide back down with a gentle stroke

hand into a fist, and lay the back of the fingers on the area of the Achilles tendon. Apply pressure to the hand by slightly bending your upper body forward, and slowly stroke upward to the hollow of the knee.

Apply deep-tissue strokes to the Achilles tendon.

• Once you are there, turn your hand at the wrist, open the fist, and gently stroke your way back to the heel with the palm of the hand. (Repeat this massage three times.)

Rubbing the calf in spiral movements

4 Hold the ankle with both your hands, so that the thumbs are placed up on the Achilles tendon while the rest of the fingers are wrapped around the leg.
• Apply pressure to the thumbs, and rub upward along the calf in small spiral movements.
• When you get to the hollow of the knee, allow your thumbs to gently glide back. Then repeat this rubbing motion two more times.

Completing the massage with strokes

5 Complete the massage on the back of the right leg by repeating Step 1 three times.

And now the left leg

6 Now switch over to the left leg, and repeat the same procedure on the opposite side.

7 In order to massage the front of the leg, your partner has to turn over now on his or her back.

Treating the front of the leg

• Start massaging the right leg, and then move over to the left leg, by repeating the grips explained in Steps 1 through 5. However, you should skip the

deep-tissue stroke explained in Step 3, because it is not possible to administer it on the shins. Also, be careful not to apply too much pressure while carrying out the movement described in Step 4.

8 You complete the leg massage with a massage grip that has the effect of removing any built-up tension:

Pressing out tension on the leg

• Hold the leg at the ankle with both hands. Apply pressure through your hands, holding the leg in place. Stroke along the inner and outer sides of the leg all the way up to the hip.
• Once you have reached the hip, let your hands gently glide back. Repeat this "pressing-out-tension stroke" two more times.

. . . and the Feet

Important: If your partner's feet are very ticklish, it's best to start the massage with a degree of firmness.

9 Spread only a few drops of oil on your hands, and hold the right foot at the heel.

Again, start on the right side.

• Apply some pressure, and stroke with both hands at the same time along the contours of the foot up toward the toes. Without diminishing the pressure, stroke back to the heel

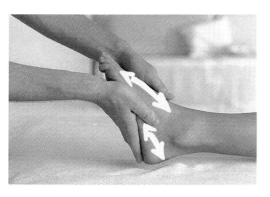

between the big toe and the toe next to it, and stroke this spot, while applying moderate pressure toward the center of the back of the foot. Be sure not to place your thumb on the bone—it should be in the area between the bones.

Do not massage the bones.

• Allow the thumbs to gently glide back to the starting position, in order to repeat the stroke three times.

• Stroke all the spaces in between the toes, to the little toe, in the same way.

Stroking the foot and then stroke upward again to the toes.

• Repeat this stroke until the massage oil is spread evenly over the entire foot.

10 The areas between the toes have reflex zones related to the upper lymph passages (see page 21), which can be stimulated intensely through deep strokes:

Stroking the area between the toes

• Support the foot on its bottom with your right hand. Lay the thumb of the left hand

11 Hold the foot with both hands, so that your thumbs are close to each other at the center of the toe-joint area. Apply pressure with both thumbs, and

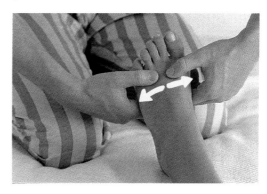

move them in opposite directions from each other—one moves toward the inner side of the foot and the other toward the outer side of the foot.

Stroking the foot to the left and to the right

• Next, place the thumbs a little

bit higher on the back of the foot, and move again from the center of the foot to the left and *Stroking* to the right.

across the • Repeat as many times as need-
entire back ed to reach the ankle.
of the foot • Once you have arrived at the ankle, allow both thumbs to gently glide back, and then repeat these opposing motions two more times.

12 The following is the "caterpillar-movement technique" to be applied on the sole of the foot:
• Stabilize the right foot with your left hand by holding the toes of the foot in place. Put the thumb of your right hand flat against the area below the joint
Press and of the small toe.
push with • Apply pressure through the
the thumb on thumb, and push it a little fur-
the sole of ther across the foot. Then bend
the foot. your thumb sharply, so that the tip of your thumb presses into

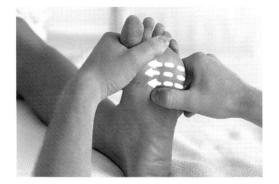

the skin and in this way creates local pressure on a specific point. Immediately afterward, let up on the pressure, allowing the thumb to lie flat again, and then push a little further. The order in which you move should be as follows: first push forward, then push inward, then push forward again. Work your way slowly across the entire foot in this manner, all the way to *Massaging* the inner side of the foot, next *the entire* to the joint of the big toe. *sole of the*
• Next, release the thumb into *foot in a* its flat lying position, and allow *"caterpillar* it to glide back to the outer side *movement."* of the foot, letting it rest a little lower than the previous spot that you treated.
• Repeat the "caterpillar-movement technique" until you have worked your way through the entire sole of the foot, from the top on down to the very bottom. By doing so, you will have massaged all the reflex zones and stimulated the circulation of the blood in the foot.

13 All the reflex zones that *Treating the* have to do with the area *head* of the head are found on the *through the* toes (see page 21): *toes*
• Hold the right foot at the heel and the ankle joint with your left hand.
• Lay the tip of your right thumb over the joint at the base

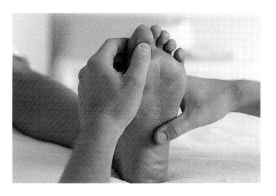

Stroking the toes one after the other of the big toe. Apply some pressure to the joint, and slowly push your thumb up toward the tip of the toe.

- Afterward, let your thumb glide back, and then repeat this upward stroke three more times.
- Repeat the same process for every single toe.

14 **Applying deep-tissue strokes to the sole of the foot** This is how you complete the foot massage:
- Hold the toes of the foot with your left hand, in order to stabilize the foot.

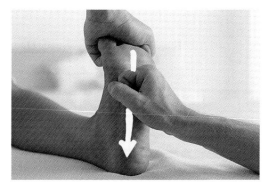

- Make a fist with your right hand, and lay the flat part on the sole of the foot, right below the joints at the base of the toes. Apply pressure with your fist, and stroke the sole of the foot down to the heel. While stroking, turn your hand a little so that the knuckles are on top. **Massaging with the knuckles of the fingers**
- When you arrive at the heel, open the fist without interrupting the continuous contact with the skin, and stroke the foot with your palm, moving back to the starting position.
- Next, quickly make your hand into a fist again, and repeat the upward strokes (three more times).

15 Following this, massage the left foot in the same manner. **Now comes the left foot's turn.**

16 After you have finished treating both feet, apply gentle pressure to the calming points on the soles of the feet: **At the end, press the calming points.**
- Place your thumbs on the center of both feet at the same time, and hold the pressure on these points for about 15 seconds.

Index

About the Author

Karin Schutt, born in 1955, has studied communications, psychology, and education, as well as breathing therapy and massage. Since 1985, she has written about various health topics.

Photos: Christian Dahl
    Further photos and illustrations: Archive of the Visual Image, Prussian Cultural Possessions, page 18; Martin Scharf, page 21, page 79 left, all arrows; Christophe Schneider, page 27, page 32; Tausendblauwerk (Michael Berwanger), page 22; Tony Stone (Howard Grey), page 15.